The Psychology of Illness

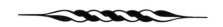

In Sickness and In Health

The Psychology of Illness

In Sickness and In Health

Richard G. Druss, M.D.

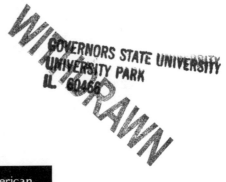

American Psychiatric Press, Inc.

Washington, DC
London, England

Copyright © 1995 American Psychiatric Press, Inc.
ALL RIGHTS RESERVED
Manufactured in the United States of America on acid-free paper
98 97 96 95   4 3 2 1
First Edition

American Psychiatric Press, Inc.
1400 K Street, N.W., Washington, DC   20005

Library of Congress Cataloging-in-Publication Data
Druss, Richard G., 1933–
    The psychology of illness : in sickness and in health / Richard G.
    Druss. — 1st ed.
        p.   cm.
    Includes bibliographical references and index.
    ISBN 0-88048-661-9 (alk. paper)
    1. Medicine and psychology. 2. Psychophysiology. I. Title.
    [DNLM: 1. Psychophysiology. 2. Psychotherapy. 3. Health
Promotion.   WL 103 D797i 1995]
    R726.5.D78   1995
    155.9′16—dc20
    DNLM/DLC
    for Library of Congress   94-23688
                                                                            CIP

British Library Cataloguing in Publication Data
A CIP record is available from the British Library.

To Margery, Benjamin, and Elizabeth

Contents

Foreword

Initiation of this foreword has presented me with an unusual delaying impediment. This impediment clearly derives from the memories of my own most threatening illness, now almost two decades in the past. I had not the slightest hesitation in responding affirmatively to the author when he inquired whether I would pen my thoughts about this book. Over many years, since he first entered this specialty of medicine, the author's professional writings on his observations of the emotional turmoil in people with physical diseases have been of particular interest to me.

Because we have known each other and have been faculty colleagues and friends throughout this time, the author remains "Dick Druss" in my mind, but I shall address him most formally here, because he has presented us with a serious work. He knows of my ileocolostomy, suddenly performed on me, that almost took me away. I have not shared with him all the complications of living with the colostomy, but he will understand my hesitancy in writing about it.

In his introduction, Dr. Druss immediately tells us that his interest in this area of psychiatric practice commenced with his very early experience in the treatment of a young woman who had suffered for years with chronic ulcerative colitis and then underwent an ileostomy. Every psychotherapist reading will now comprehend the reason for my initial impediment. Now we shall put that aside.

In the course of his treatment of this woman, Dr. Druss came to recognize that her image of her body underwent a change. His treatment used a psychodynamic technique that provided him with valuable insights and information about the early development of his patient. This rewarding clinical experience, which led to an excellent living adaptation for his patient, whetted his curiosity, to which he applied all that drive and energy that he has applied not only to patients with ulcerative colitis but also to patients who underwent required or elective surgical and medical procedures, examining in each group the changes that took place in their body image and in the nuclear aspect of their self-concept. Thus, he has written about and published his observations of those who have lived on after ileostomy, colostomy, mastectomy, and augmentation breast surgery as well as those with cryptorchidism and the drive for perfectionism in anorexia. With this unusual and wide clinical experience, a book from Dr. Druss surely promises further insights.

And so it does provide them.

Dr. Druss has probed the personalities of those who have suffered or experienced the consequences and outcomes over time of both medical and surgical interventions. Struck by the unusual resilience of some people in overcoming their enduring handicaps and their demonstrated capacity to continue long, active, and productive lives, he went beyond his own observations to autobiographical and biographical writings to search for the beginnings of those character traits from which their strengths seemed to derive. He provides interpretations of both sickness- and health-driven behaviors with striking clinical descriptions. Thus, in some ill people, he has found that denial sustained sickness behavior. But Dr. Druss notes the paradox that "healthy denial" is a fulcrum for many who have made extraordinary adaptations to life in the course of unusual and persisting symptomatic expression.

In light of what you have already learned about this book, it shall come as no surprise that Dr. Druss's treatment philosophy is presented as founded on empathy, flexibility, the historical perspective, and an attitude of therapeutic optimism. Each of the sections in Chapter 5, "Treatment Philosophy," is important reading for those who work with medically ill patients. I commend particularly the section on flexibility, wherein Dr. Druss demonstrates his willingness both to modify his general psychodynamic stance and to recommend pharmacological interventions for some, as well as insights and support to be achieved by patients' participation in the various group therapies now available. Nor is the final section on optimism to be overlooked. He ends it by noting that "psychiatrists treating medically ill patients must manifest their optimism, not about the patient's course or ultimate prognosis, which no one knows, but about the patient's courage, no matter what the outcome."

Dr. Druss then immerses his reader in that continuing entrancing mystery and search for the sources of strength that provide the psychological structure for one to endure and live constructively in the face of illness and disability. This is *health*. As he reflects on those whom he has treated as well as others he has come to know through their biographies, one is brought to consider with him that more is demanded in explanation than references to their psychological defenses. With others who have studied the eminently successful, he finds it necessary to go beyond the traditional psychoanalytic interpretations of character structure based on defensive traits.

Dr. Druss looks to the life of fantasy into which so many isolated chronically ill people spend their time as one resource from which their strength emerges. This is wonderfully illustrated in his discussion of the life of Robert Louis Stevenson, whose stories entertained and even today entertain so many. Here commences his search for the development of those character traits he considers important in finding health in illness. The source of those personality traits that betoken the healthy response to the trauma of illness he has found in his patients' identification with parents and role models who encouraged and rewarded robustness, exuberance, and self-reliance.

The Psychology of Illness: In Sickness and In Health organizes the clinical inferences that we psychiatrists may derive from the clinical data received from their medically ill patients. It also brings us to search for and support by all available means those personality assets that will make possible for each patient a more healthy life adaptation. Even more significant to me are the questions raised about our knowledge base and theoretical positions in regard to personality and personality structure.

Once again, we find in these pages the evidence that too little has been given to developmental research and insufficient emphasis has been laid on those rewarding transactions in growth that, integrated with our defensive structure, provide the true foundations of mental health.

Lawrence C. Kolb, M.D.

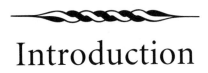

Introduction

As I write this, the federal health program is still evolving, and every citizen will have to adjust to major changes in his or her health care. No matter what the outcome, and how secure their pocketbook may be, people will continue to get sick and be frightened about their sickness. And no matter what the outcome, there will be a need for psychiatrists to consult with and treat many of these medically ill patients. The chronically ill can be a neglected group, often left bewildered and overwhelmed. The psychiatrist has the opportunity to help patients cope not only with their illness but with the increasingly complex relationship with their physician and the medical establishment. As the population ages, and as sicker people live longer, there is an increasing need for someone to accompany chronically ill patients on their difficult journey through illness. I believe that as psychiatrists it is often our role to be that companion; we are privileged to have both the medical and the psychological training. All one needs is a willingness to take on these worthwhile patients—and a guide. And it is for that reason that I have written this book.

In the spring of my second year of training at the College of Physicians & Surgeons of Columbia University, I evaluated an intelligent young woman of 20 who had serious ulcerative colitis and was prepared to undertake a year of psychodynamic psychotherapy starting after Labor Day. Then, as fate would have it, she had an exacerbation of her disease and underwent an emergency removal of her colon that summer. When Labor Day rolled around, she no longer had a "classical psychosomatic" disorder but was struggling to cope with a new, permanent ileostomy.

In addition to conducting a standard psychodynamic psychotherapy, I spent the next year being educated firsthand about life with an ileostomy. My patient said she was happy that without her diseased colon she was no longer a "prisoner of the bathroom," having to plot her daily activities according to the availability and location of rest rooms. She was also no longer anemic and perpetually fatigued and could finally discontinue steroids, with their numerous unpleasant side effects. But in the course of her therapy, she recounted the downside as well. She spoke with some shame about defecating without control from an opening in her abdomen into a bag that requires daily hygiene and changing. She described the embarrassment over unexpected noises and smells, and the special requirements of her diet. The sessions focused on her concern that she would not be cosmetically acceptable to a future boyfriend or husband. She was openly angry at the failure of the medical profession to be of much help. She felt that the surgeons cut and ran, that the internists and nurses had little practical information on ileostomy care, and that we psychiatrists were vastly more interested in entities we could try to "cure," such as active colitis, rather than "failures" who ended up without their colons. The scanty medical and psychiatric literature about ileostomy at that time supported her viewpoint.

One savior turned out to be the Ileostomy Club in New York City. This self-help group was one of several modeled after Alcoholics Anonymous that sprang up to fill the gap left by medical science. They discussed the nitty-gritty of the everyday life of the ileostomy patient—everything from the latest adhesive gum to attach the ileostomy container, to diet and local skin care, to social and sexual etiquette. Equally important, they offer support, knowledge gained by experience, and a place for regular socialization. Self-help groups for people with specific diseases, now commonplace for even rare medical conditions, were uncommon in 1965. My patient invited me to attend some of the club meetings as an observer, which I did.

Much of our psychotherapeutic work also dealt with the patient's adjustment to a new body image. The ileostomy derived from her small intestine was a phallic-shaped lower abdominal organ and was responsive to changes in mood and blood flow. She had to integrate and accept this new organ within an overall feminine orientation.

It was a productive year for both of us, and it led me toward a lifetime path of research into and writing about the effects of various sorts of changes in the body on mental life. Here is where I parted company with many of my psychoanalytic colleagues who remained interested in the psychogenesis of physical disorders. (By the way, the patient did well, married, and sent me announcements in the succeeding years of the births of their three children.)

During the last 9 years, I have conducted a weekly seminar for PGY-II residents and staff at a medical-psychiatric unit at Columbia-Presbyterian Hospital. Every other week, we discuss a patient who has a medical disorder and psychiatric problems. On alternate weeks, I assign a piece of popular literature, classical or contemporary (as opposed to a journal article), that illuminates the subjective experience of being sick, and we discuss it together. This experience keeps me on my toes and often led quite directly to the chapters that follow. Bright, skeptical, and enthusiastic residents have become my current teachers.

The first half of the book is devoted to sickness and what it means to be sick. Chapter 1 is composed of a series of excerpts from some of the autobiographical selections discussed in the seminars. They are by talented authors who write openly and movingly about their experiences as patients. The choices were made with care, and each is from a classic that I recommend reading in its entirety.

Chapter 2 is on hypochondriasis as it appears in people who are already ill. Some chronically ill people suffer the added burden of excessive anxiety about the course and outcome of their illness or about some necessary diagnostic or therapeutic procedure. After reviewing some of the literature on hypochondriasis, I present three case reports and then offer a hypothesis about why some sick people worry so much.

In Chapter 3, I cover pathological denial. Denial of illness can be truly self-destructive, and this chapter addresses this defense mechanism seen commonly in consultation-liaison psychiatry. I present vignettes of two rather extreme cases that spell out the problem in headlines. Then I finish with a section on denial in everyday life, equally important and seen to some extent in most people, but all too rarely addressed by physicians.

Next, I present two chapters on treatment. Chapter 4 is a lengthy case history of a patient recovering from a malignancy who was treated with psychodynamic psychotherapy. I feel there is still a place for the richness of detail that can only be seen in the report of the process of a treatment. I also hope to demonstrate that for a selected few, an in-depth psychodynamic psychotherapy can be the treatment of choice.

At the end of this section is Chapter 5, on the broader spectrum of psychiatric treatments for medically ill patients. I discuss cognitive and behavior therapies, psychopharmacological therapy, couples and family therapies, hospital visits and telephone sessions to preserve treatment continuity, and the use of self-help groups. The chapter is truly multidisciplinary in scope.

The second section of the book is on health and staying healthy. I hold that this is an area often neglected in the usual training of physicians and other healers. Yet the public is bombarded by the media with advice on health care and prevention of illness, and we should be no less well-equipped to deal authoritatively with these subjects. Our patients will ask us about keeping fit, and we should have answers and programs. Some of the newer data on "alternative medicine" are included in this section.

The first chapter in this section, Chapter 6, is on healthy denial. The very fact that denial can be healthy is a paradox that I explore in depth. The chapter deals with a whole range of positive adaptations to illness that can be powerful tools when properly used. Three very different case vignettes are presented and discussed.

Chapter 7 is on courage. Courage facing chronic illness is a theme that reappears throughout the book, residing as it does somewhere between clinical psychiatry and philosophy, but this chapter focuses on it. The "clinical case" material is from the life of Robert Louis Stevenson, a writer racked by severe tuberculosis all of his life, yet who showed great courage.

The final chapter, Chapter 8, is on the positive steps one can take toward maintaining health or maintaining a healthy attitude when ill. It deals with exercise, fitness, and that elusive entity "quality of life," sick or well.

In each chapter, I have attempted to address the subjective experience of what it means to be chronically ill. The reader will find many clinical accounts, some consistent theory derived from them, up-to-date references, and 25 years of experience that I hope to share with beginners in psychiatry: medical students, residents, and fellows. But the book is written with a wider audience in mind. It is addressed to all those who tend the sick: primary care physicians, psychologists, nurses, social workers, physical and occupational therapists, and pastoral counselors of all faiths.

Writing a single-author book is not a solo task, and I acknowledge the vast help of a few people who made it possible. First, I thank Dr. Carol Nadelson, Editor-in-Chief of the American Psychiatric Press, Inc., for her encouragement and faith in this project and for her suggestions, which were always on the mark. Second, I thank Claire Reinburg, Editorial Director, who has been my Virgil, leading me through the mysterious world of book writing, always helpful, always reassuring. Third, I thank Pamela Harley, Managing Editor, for transforming all of this into a palpable reality.

At my end, I owe much gratitude to Dr. Carolyn Douglas, Chief of the Psychiatric-Medical Unit on which I consulted. She is coauthor of two articles on denial from which the two chapters on denial in this book are derived. Dr. Douglas and Dr. Jennifer Downy were both kind and long suffering enough to read the entire manuscript, as did four residents in our program, Drs. Adrienne Birt, Michael Kaplan, Justine Kent, and Ze'ev Levin.

Other colleagues read various chapters in earlier incarnations and offered invaluable help: Drs. Milton Viederman, Ethel Person, Willard Gaylin, Arnold Cooper, Gerald Fogel, Hillary Beattie, and the late Robert Liebert. Special thanks are due to Jonathan Jackson, who decoded my hen scratches and typed them into words; I'm still a creature of the pen and yellow pad era. I am grateful to Judy Kronenberg for her expert library skills.

I am honored that Dr. Lawrence C. Kolb consented to write a foreword to this volume. A true healer, he taught, by word and example, that the patient always comes first.

My children, Benjamin and Elizabeth, both young physicians-in-training, were merciless in their loving criticism of the manuscript and made sure my attitudes and consciousness were as up-to-date as my references. Finally, my wife, Margery, gave her continuing devotion, encouragement, and love for this project and to me.

About the Author

Richard G. Druss, M.D., is Clinical Professor of Psychiatry at the College of Physicians & Surgeons of Columbia University. He is the immediate past Associate Director of the Columbia University Psychoanalytic Center for Training and Research.

I

Sickness

1

~~~~~~~~~~~~~~~

Illness as Depicted in Popular Literature

Shortly before he died of dissemi-nated cancer, Anatole Broyard wrote a book, *Intoxicated by My Illness* (1992), in which he said, "A critical illness is one of our momentous experiences, yet I haven't seen a single nonfiction book that does it justice" (p. 13). I disagree.

During the last 9 years, I have been teaching a seminar to beginning psychiatry residents at the College of Physicians & Surgeons of Columbia University on the subjective aspects of illness—that is, from the point of view of the patient rather than of the physician. We use literature, mainly autobiographical accounts, as the vehicle to achieve this goal.

As therapists, we are obliged to take a special interest in the subjective experience of medically ill patients, and here the scientific literature often fails us. What is written by objective observers misses the inner life of those who are afflicted.

In recent years, a large number of books and memoirs have been pub-lished by patients and former patients in which these persons describe their own experiences with sickness. We live in a confessional age, and what was formerly taboo is now exhibited freely. This popular (as opposed to profes-sional) literature, however, offers a window into the world of the ill. All of the books I cite can be commended to the reader on their own merits. Although it has limitations in terms of both methodology and content, "non-scientific" literature provides us with an additional and unique vantage point into the psychology of illness.

Problems of Chronic Illness

Six common problems emerge on reading these books, and they parallel those present in the narratives of my own medically ill patients. The list of problems is arbitrary, with many overlapping themes—but it is a start: 1) illness as punishment leading to unlovability, 2) illness leading to a state of helplessness, 3) illness involving a sense of betrayal, 4) illness causing changes in the self, 5) illness becoming a preoccupation, and 6) illness as a cause of loss. I take these in turn and then discuss some of the factors that make for a good psychological prognosis and lead to successful coping mechanisms.

Illness as Punishment Leading to a Sense of Unlovability

Illness as punishment leading to a sense of unlovability is an old idea that goes back as far as the Hebrew Bible. Job's Comforters feel that in a just world Job would not suffer such misfortunes unless they were deserved. By the time of the advent of Christianity, illness had come to be regarded as divine punishment for the commission of sins, both the hidden and the revealed (Sontag 1979). Many victims of catastrophe regard any of life's tragedies as fair punishment for known or unknown past iniquities. Many patients do not participate or cooperate in the fight against their illness because of a conviction that they deserve it. These are individuals with the fertile soil of free-floating guilt who lie waiting for an event worthy of pinning it on. Their crimes are the foibles, instincts, and drives of all individuals and go back to early childhood: anger at a rival, illicit sexual cravings, petty selfish outlook, refusal to obey, or omission of a law, rule, or obligation. This view reflects a harsh superego that has accumulated a list of petty infractions and venial sins. It is the thoughts that seem to require punishment—murder, incest, devouring—none of which are conscious to the individual.

Depression often accompanies chronic illness and is one of the most common reasons for psychiatric intervention (Viederman and Perry 1980).

Depression, unlike grief, is a maladaptive response to the crisis of illness. The depression is characterized by a generalized lowering of self-esteem, by irrational guilt and self-accusations, and by a state of hopelessness that is quite beyond the restrictions posed by the illness. But in addition to depression, when a serious illness strikes, the patient feels punished and, by extension, unloved by the punisher. The feeling of being unloved, and unlovable, is one of the signal hallmarks of chronic illness. In 1970, when I began my 7-year position as consultant to the Plastic Surgery Service at Presbyterian Hospital, I recall being enormously impressed that its director of service would embrace his ongoing patients who returned for their periodic clinic visits. His embrace of these individuals with dreadful facial anomalies, inoperable lymphangiomas, bladder extrophies, etc., did much to make them feel worthwhile and was worth more than words alone. I further recall, at a study group of the American Psychoanalytic Association, the late Dr. Norman R. Bernstein's admonitions regarding the care of severe burn victims: to hold physically an unaffected part—a toe, or ear, or hand—during one's bedside interview; and Dr. Lawrence Kolb's equally important advice for psychiatrists engaged in liaison work: to look at the amputation stump, scar, ileostomy, etc., and, by looking, to accept it.

Arthur Kleinman, in *The Illness Narratives* (1988), described patients who have influenced his career:

> The first patient was a pathetic 7-year-old girl who had been badly burned over most of her body. She had to undergo a daily ordeal of a whirlpool bath during which the burnt flesh was tweezered away from her raw open wounds. The experience was horribly painful to her. Clumsily, with a beginner's uncertainty of how to proceed, I tried to distract this little patient from her traumatic daily confrontation with terrible pain. I tried talking to her about her home, her family, her school, almost anything that might draw her vigilant attention away from her suffering. I could barely tolerate the daily horror: her screams, dead tissue floating in the blood-stained water, the peeling flesh, the oozing wounds, the battles over cleaning and bandaging. Then one day I made contact. At wit's end, angered by my own ignorance, uncertain what to do besides clutching the small hand, I found myself asking her how she tolerated it. She stopped, quite surprised; then in terms direct and simple she told me. While she spoke, she grasped my hand harder and neither fought off the surgeon or the nurse. Each day from then on, her trust established, she tried to give me a feeling of what she was experiencing. (p. xi)

All of these tactile visual techniques address the physical sense of deficit. The patient feels like an unlovable child who has been punished, and it is this dreadful self-appraisal that adds to the misery of illness. Psychiatrists in office practice are usually not afforded the opportunity of looking at or touching the lesions of medically ill people but nonetheless have to convey their acceptance by openly addressing these issues.

Because so much of the sufferings of people with medical illness are caused by disturbances of physical function, I wish to elaborate on the importance of nonverbal adjunctive treatments. The ancient attribute of physicians in the laying on of hands was a precious part of their healing armamentarium. Yet there are other professions that may attend to these needs better than physicians. I recall one of my medical professors at Columbia, Dr. Yale Kneeland, that supreme internist, saying to his surprised group of medical students that should he become ill and have the choice of the world's best nurse and a fair internist, or the world's best internist and a mediocre nurse, he would surely choose the former. Many patients would benefit from physical therapy, massage, and good bedside nursing because their bodies ache for physical contact. Eminent biophysicist Dr. Frederick Sachs, writing in *The Sciences* (1988), said,

> The fundamental nature of touch is even more apparent when the sense is deprived of stimulation. Being unable to hear or see does not prevent one from attaining a happy or fruitful existence; countless deaf or blind people overcome the difficulties imposed by their handicaps and live otherwise normal lives. But an existence devoid of tactile sensation is another matter; sustained physical contact with other human beings is a prerequisite for healthy relationships and for successful engagement with the rest of one's environment. Denial of physical contact during the first years of life can cause virtually irreversible states of withdrawal. Touch, in short, is the core of sentience, the foundation for communication with the world around us, and probably the single sense that is as old as life itself. (p. 28)

Society does not help and has its own similar practices. The sick person is quarantined like the patient with diphtheria, cast out like the leper, shunned like the person with AIDS. Even in modern, enlightened hospitals, the terminally ill patients are put aside, skipped on rounds, and hidden from view. They are the untouchable caste and to be avoided lest one be tainted by association. No wonder they feel unloved.

Illness Leading to a State of Helplessness

The regressive aspects of illness are legion. Disease is experienced as humiliating and demeaning as well as unpleasant. The loss of control, the taking away of status and position in the hospital, all contribute to the sense of helplessness. In the book *Risk* (1990), written about the dehumanizing experience of being hospitalized, Rachael MacKenzie describes her own open-heart surgery. This well-regarded editor at *The New Yorker* takes the reader into the minute details of her experience and, in less than 100 pages, makes us witness to them. She uses the third person and begins her book thusly (p. 3):

> "I think it's time you saw a super-super heart man," Dr. Lewis said. "You recall, I told you I might want you to. We'll make the arrangements and be in touch."
>
> The appointment with Dr. Jamison was on January 13th. "I have your recent hospital record," he said when she called from the office where she worked, "and I've talked with Dr. Lewis and have his recent cardiogram and X rays and I guess that's everything I need."
>
> "Except me," she said.

Humankind's struggle is toward greater independence and individuation, greater mastery and control. Illness, insofar as it mimics the helplessness of childhood, exerts its regressive pull. The writers who succeeded in their quest to get better maintained some level of control over their circumstances. They demanded to be full partners of the physician rather than helpless children. The dread of helplessness and regression to a former loathed state of dependency where sureness of care is uncertain was a universal accompaniment of chronic illness. Each individual has a secret fantasy of the end point of that illness—for some it is to become very ugly and repellent, for some to be alone, for others to be racked with pain—for this group it is a state of helplessness, dependent on others, humiliated and ashamed.

Richard Rovere, the late political commentator and biographer of Senator Joseph McCarthy, developed a malignancy deep in his neck that caused him constant pain. He wrote at the end of his collection of essays, *Final Reports* (1984):

> Oh, but I hate it, hate it, hate it. I hate it and fear it and can find few words that reach the depths of my feeling. The truth is that my character is being

altered in ways I find unbearable to record. I seem to myself to become pettier and meaner and more selfish by the hour. (p. 228)

For those for whom dependency was loathsome, who couldn't grow up fast enough, the fear is enough, and the anticipation demoralizing. Every aspect of illness conspires to place the ill person in a dependent position: pain, fear, limitations of function. What enables some to overcome the regressive pull? When the realities are overwhelming, no one can remain untouched. For example, virtually everyone landing at Omaha Beach on D day was shattered by the physical dangers and deprivations. But each symptom has its symbolic representations and touches primitive fears—of castration, engulfment, dissolution of self. It is the special province of psychotherapy to unearth the neurotic infrastructure of physical symptoms and their uniqueness to that person's past. For some whose face is their fortune, a skin lesion would terrify them more than it might others; for others for whom mobility is necessary, bed rest, paralysis, or even a limp becomes their Achilles' heel.

Norman Cousins, former editor of *The Saturday Review,* documents his own heart attack vividly in *The Healing Heart* (1983). Where did he learn that he could be an equal partner with his physician and be able to demand this right even when in the middle of a coronary occlusion?

Betty Rollin, a television reporter herself working on a documentary on breast cancer, underwent a mastectomy. In *First You Cry* (1976), she gives hints on how she overcame the pull of regression. Her mother said to the nurse, "My daughter is a fighter," and Rollin said of her mother, "Her spunk was magnificent." The devotion for and identification with a brave mother is clear. She learned courage at her mother's knee, and her fighting spirit was valued by her mother.

We see a counterphobic tone in both Rollin's and Cousins's books. Rollin, describing her mastectomy, tells everyone that she had a "breast cut off for cancer," and she enjoyed shocking stuffy dinner partners with such openers. Perhaps to acquire mastery over regression one must begin with some bravado to avoid the shame of silence and secrets, even when it offends or discomforts others or overshoots the mark.

Illness as a Betrayal

The third consequence of chronic illness is a sense of narcissistic betrayal. Perfectionist individuals demanding bodily perfection do badly with any illness or even the aging process. A horrifying recollection is the woman with breast cancer who conducted a public presuicide party on a recent public television program rather than undergo what would have likely been a curative mastectomy. The stated view was that she was "unwilling to live the imperfect life."

In addition, these individuals say to themselves, "Why me?" They are angry at everyone, angry at the diagnostician for discovering the disease, angry at the surgeon for mutilating them, and angry at the radiotherapist or oncologist for the continuance of their disability and the side effects of treatments. They are angry at the people around them, family and friends, envying others' good health. They have the conviction that they "signed a contract" in childhood that if only they would be good then life would offer them no bad news. When illness comes, they feel betrayed, repeating the betrayal of very early losses and traumas.

This sense of betrayal, when coupled with the regression previously discussed, can lead to powerful transferences toward the physician. The physician can be the messenger of bad tidings who must tell the patient, "Nothing can be done," or "There is a recurrence," and the messenger can be hated for his or her message. In addition, the kind of magical thinking operative in these patients leads to the expectation that the doctor should be able to fix anything and would do so if he or she really wanted to. These feelings are universal, but in most patients they are transient, and an adult observing-ego ultimately prevails.

Walter W. Benjamin wrote in the essay "Healing by the Fundamentals" (1986),

> A friend of mine is dying of lupus at the age of 40. . . . Her anger at not being able to see her children marry is intense; how unfair life is! Her anger zeroed in on her physician, even though, because of drug sensitivity, his therapeutic choices were limited. Once, as she was attacking him for the absurdity of her fate, she saw a tear in his eye. "All my anger dissolved in a minute, for I knew he cared," she said. . . . No longer adversaries, they had become two human beings sharing tragedy together. (p. 595)

The key word is *sharing*, which opposes the infantilization of the patient, lessens the expectations, and reduces the sense that he or she has been a victim of betrayal. Broyard (1992) said it well:

What a critically ill person needs above all is to be understood. Dying is a misunderstanding you have to get straightened out before you go. And you can't be understood, your situation can't be appreciated, until your family and friends, staring at you with an embarrassed love, come to know with an intimate, absolute knowledge, what your illness is like. (p. 67)

Illness and Alteration in the Self

I conducted a study of healthy women who decided to undergo augmentation breast surgery (Druss 1973). These women reported a period of private tactile exploration of their new breasts after the surgery. Slowly, the implant, producing sensation in the chest wall *and* the hand, became integrated as a part of them, rather than a foreign body.

A reverse intrapsychic process occurs during the accommodation to chronic illness. The boundaries of the self must be reduced, and the sickness must be viewed as external to one's essence rather than as a part of the self. Chronically ill patients have to believe that they are uninjured and that the battle between the disease and a drug or surgery occurs outside some central core self, which remains inviolable.

This attitude is most obvious in a condition like breast cancer. Rollin (1976) described her denial, overcompensation, and exhibitionism after her mastectomy. But then, after mourning for the lost organ, she stated that *she* has not changed in some fundamental way; she is the same, and it is only a sick breast that has been removed.

This approach may be less effective when the diseased organ is central to life (such as the heart or brain) or the illness is disseminated in a widespread infection, immunodeficiency, or metastasized cancer. Nonetheless, the individual avers something like, "They can have my leg or heart or strength, but they can't have me." The attack can reach the perimeter, which may have to be sacrificed, but the soul or the central core remains intact. Prisoners of war and Holocaust survivors have reported a similar state of mind.

One of the consequences of this adaptive shrinkage of boundaries is a turning within and a heightening of fantasy during crises and reversals (such as in the writings of Robert Louis Stevenson, discussed in Chapter 7). Although people are more willing or able to write about the resilient or heroic aspects of their coping than about the entry into their narrowed private space, many of the books are remarkable in their honesty describing it.

Illness as a Preoccupation

Chronic illness has the capacity to become a central focus of an individual's life by its realistic intrusions. Chronic illness is hard to ignore and reminds us of our bodily entrapment. Illness can become a psychological preoccupation as well, allowing little conflict-free ego to attend to other matters. The patient with ulcerative colitis must arrange his or her daily path with the location of bathroom facilities known in advance because the need will and does arise often and suddenly. The person with brittle diabetes must know before any trip or vacation where a trusted medical facility is. The wheelchair-bound person must know in elaborate and boring detail about such mundane matters as steps and revolving doors.

John Updike wrote about his psoriasis in "At War With My Skin," a remarkably honest confession in his book *Self-Consciousness* (1989),

> Because of my skin I counted myself out of any of these jobs—salesman, teacher, financier, movie star—that demand being presentable. What did that leave? Becoming a craftsman of some sort, closeted and unseen—perhaps a cartoonist or a writer: a worker in ink who can hide himself and send out a surrogate presence, a signature that multiplies while it conceals. . . . Why did I leave New York and my snug apartment there? Because my skin was bad in the urban shadows. . . . Why did I move with my family to Ipswich, Massachusetts? Because this ancient Puritan town happened to have one of the great beaches in the Northeast. . . . From April to November my life was structured around giving my skin a dose of sun. (pp. 48ff)

Updike goes to the Caribbean each winter in search of year-round sun. He then enrolls at the Massachusetts General psoriasis ultraviolet light program, still in the experimental stage. He described a humiliating exposure:

> When I broke my leg and had to have it operated upon, I chiefly remember being pleased that my shins, in that season, were clear and that I would not offend the surgeon. (p. 76)

Steve Fishman is a young journalist in excellent health who had a catastrophic rupture of an arterial malformation in his brain. In *A Bomb in the Brain* (1988), he described a degree of preoccupation with his condition that became in his own terms "an obsession." After neurosurgery, he devoured medical texts, attended neurology conferences, trailed residents, and observed brain surgery. After the otherwise successful surgery, he developed a chronic seizure disorder that perpetuated his obsession. An intimate relationship with a woman ended because his thoughts and attention were totally consumed by his medical condition. He said at the end of his preface, "If this is a story of a career in neurosurgery, it is mine" (p. xiv).

The difficult point for anyone with such a disorder is knowing how far to go with its treatment. When should one pursue the next consultation, the newest test, the latest remedy, and when should one quit and attempt to enjoy life with the limitation? This is the crucial difference from an acute or even terminal disease where one can wage, must wage, an all-out attack. Every chronic illness, like the psoriasis of Updike or the epilepsy of Fishman, has the potential for becoming a lifelong preoccupation.

Illnesses that are progressive and that cause deterioration over time induce special problems. There is no steady state or equilibrium. They always interrupt.

Illness as a Cause of Loss

Illness is poorly handled when it involves a change from better to worse and a *loss* ensues. A man born deaf who at age 40 has 20% of normal hearing restored by modern surgical techniques is perpetually grateful. Another man who at age 40 loses 80% of normal hearing and arrives at the same end point may suffer an inconsolable loss. Therefore, paradoxically, people with severe congenital deformities may do well with surgical intervention. In the account of *Lisa H.*, by Richard Severo (1985), a girl with congenital neurofibromatosis (elephant man's disease) responded well to the surgery that turned her from a hideous and grotesque young woman to just plain very ugly.

Lisa described the events of a recent Halloween to the reporter. She knew all the neighbors who had come by trick-or-treating and welcomed them; she then went to the kitchen to get the children their candy. When she returned to the living room, a longtime neighbor pointed at Lisa and chuckled, "Boy isn't that a skit? Look at that scary mask!" As he left, he was pleased that he could share an amusing moment with his son. She said she knew she could never be beautiful. She only sought to be plain enough to be left alone, to be not so different that people would recoil from the sight of her, as illustrated below (p. 8):

> "What advantages do you think you'll get out of the surgery?"
> "Well, I don't think I'm going to look like Farrah Fawcet. But I'd want the surgery if there were only 1% improvement."
> "One percent. You are taking great risks for 1%?"
> "Yes. I realize my face might be permanently paralyzed if they cut the wrong nerves."
> "What will you do if there is some paralysis?"
> "No problem. It beats looking like this."

Contrast Lisa to patients currently involved in malpractice suits because they are dissatisfied with minor scarring following a face-lift. Also, I have changed my mind about reconstructive breast surgery after mastectomy. I used to feel that immediate reconstruction was a procedure that would save the patient a year or more of misery. Numerous consultations with these women have demonstrated to me that those who wait are often more content with their reconstructed breast. Their change has been from an absent breast to a reconstructed one, rather than from a whole breast to the reconstructed one in the immediate surgical operations. Gain is always preferable to loss.

Solutions to the Problems of Chronic Illness

Individuals who are successful in coping with chronic illness often have a number of common elements in their backgrounds. First, they had as role models parents who admired robustness and self-reliance in themselves and reinforced these qualities in their children. Second, they were not spoiled. They were tested throughout their lives and had the experience of overcoming many defeats and disappointments. Finally, they did not live with the expectation of a perfect life, a life that would be forever free of pain and unhappiness if only they were good. They had little narcissistic entitlement and little narcissistic perfectionism. These characteristics enabled this group of patients to handle illness well, to cooperate in their rehabilitation, or, if doomed to die, to live their allotted days with some tranquility and then to die a good death.

One program for a successful solution to the problems of chronic illness is depicted in *Heading Home,* by Paul Tsongas (1984). He was 43, a senator from Massachusetts with a promising career, when he was diagnosed with a serious malignant condition with an uncertain but negative prognosis. It was not immediately life threatening, but there was no known cure, and the life expectancy was about 8 years. He left a successful career in politics and returned to private life as a private citizen, husband, and father. He demonstrated flexibility and the ability to make a dramatic change in his life trajectory. He underwent a reordering of priorities that so many individuals with similar illnesses seem incapable of doing. Also, as he says, he was blessed with an intelligent and supportive family, and he further stated that when his supply of strength was deficient his wife's was not. His wife, Niki, shines through the entire book. When he called her with the diagnosis, she said, "Well, we're just going to beat it, that's all, come on home" (p. 30). The disease was handled as a family team effort throughout.

Oliver Sacks, professor of neurology at Albert Einstein College of Medicine, came to his resolution by an entirely different route, described in *A Leg to Stand On* (1984). While climbing a mountain alone in Norway, he fell and injured his leg. He required surgery and was left with a flaccid paralysis of his leg. He also had a disturbance of his body image in which the limb felt as if it were not part of him, and he was therefore unable to walk. Rather than make use of family and friends, he essentially cured himself as he had hiked—alone. The curative process he described in his unique, eloquent manner was internal and almost mystical, with music playing a crucial role in the process. Tsongas was a politician and a man of the people. Sacks was private and inner directed; he said, "The solution to walking is walking. . . . The only way to do it is—to do it. The key to this paradox is the mystery of Grace. Here action and thought reach their end and repose" (p. 150).

A totally different approach is described by Alice Trillin, an educational consultant for a public television station who had a pulmonary lobectomy at age 38. She described her own method of coping with lung cancer in *Of Dragons and Garden Peas* (1981):

> One of the ways that all of us avoid thinking about death is by concentrating on the details of our daily lives. The work we do every day and the people we love—the fabric of our lives—convince us that we are alive and that we will

stay alive. . . . A year after I had my lung removed, my doctors asked me what I cared about most . . . and I told them what was most important to me was garden peas . . . that I could think of when to plant them and how much mulch they would need instead of thinking about platelets and white cells. I cherish the privilege of thinking about trivia. (p. 699)

Trillin immersed herself in the tasks of everyday life.

No discussion of coping mechanisms would be complete without some mention of the role of religion in people's lives. Paul Wilkes described this clearly in his wonderful book *In Mysterious Ways* (1990). He met Father Joseph Greer in 1987 when he asked the Archdiocese of Boston to put him into contact with a priest suffering from a life-threatening illness. Wilkes won the confidence of Father Greer, a most appealing, tough, witty, street-smart priest of the old school, who was receiving chemotherapy for multiple myeloma. Father Greer confided to Wilkes:

We priests talk humility, but a kind of arrogance is closer to the truth. Suddenly I know what it was like to be in a hospital bed, sure the doctors weren't telling you everything. Suddenly I realized Joe Greer wasn't in charge anymore. I had already faced the fact that the world wasn't black and white and that Father didn't have all the answers. But the illness made me aware of the fragility, the impermanence of all of us. It made me appreciate the Sacrament of the Sick and what a beautiful stepping-stone it is—either back to healthy life or one to the next life. Having received it myself, I can understand its power. That's why I want it for others and want them to understand what it is. It's not the closing of the coffin; it's that stepping-stone. After a year and a half on the medication, they told me there is no trace of my disease; I'm clear. But it's not really gone, and I know that. Impermanence, all over again.

So I stopped trying to bargain with God. I don't try to be any different, or look more holy than I ever was—which is not all that holy, believe me. If I have anything, it comes out in my humanity and in my work, not out of my mouth.

I just said to God I'd try to be the best priest I could if I had any time left. He gave me that time. (p. 71)

Each person has his or her own way to cope with and master chronic illness—Father Greer, Trillin, Sacks, and Tsongas. Therapists must respect each pathway, regardless of their own theoretical orientation or belief system.

The search for a good psychological outcome is the search for quality of life. It will not be found by trying to fit a patient into the therapist's therapeutic modality but by helping each patient find his or her own pathway. Self-discovery is what psychotherapy is all about, and the psychiatrist is the Socratic midwife in that search.

References

Benjamin WW: Healing by the fundamentals. N Engl J Med 311:595–597, 1986

Broyard A: Intoxicated by My Illness. New York, Clarkson Potter, 1992

Cousins N: The Healing Heart. New York, WW Norton, 1983

Druss RG: Changes in body image following augmentation breast surgery. International Journal of Psychoanalysis and Psychotherapy 2:248–256, 1973

Fishman S: A Bomb in the Brain. New York, Charles Scribner, 1988

Kleinman A: The Illness Narratives: Suffering, Healing, and the Human Condition. New York, Basic Books, 1988

MacKenzie R: Risk. New York, Viking, 1990

Rollin B: First You Cry. New York, Signet, 1976

Rovere R: Final Reports. New York, Doubleday, 1984

Sachs F: The intimate sense. The Sciences 28:28–34, 1988

Sacks O: A Leg to Stand On. New York, Summit, 1984

Severo R: Lisa H. New York, Harper & Row, 1985

Sontag S: Illness as Metaphor. New York, Vintage, 1979

Trillin A: Of dragons and garden peas. N Engl J Med 304:699, 1981

Tsongas P: Heading Home. New York, Alfred A Knopf, 1984

Updike J: At war with my skin, in Self-Consciousness. New York, Alfred A Knopf, 1989, pp 42–78

Viederman M, Perry S: Use of psychodynamic life narrative in the treatment of depression in the physically ill. Gen Hosp Psychiatry 3:177–185, 1980

Wilkes P: In Mysterious Ways: The Death and Life of a Parish Priest. New York, Random House, 1990

2

Hypochondriasis in Medically Ill Patients

Chronically ill people are doubly cursed. Not only do they have a physical illness, but they can be burdened by excessive worry, preoccupation, and pessimism about it. I devote this chapter to those individuals who *are* ill but who are handling their condition with overconcern, morbid ideation, and anxiety that may approach panic. When their anxious concern is fairly brief, less than 6 months, we would classify these patients as having an adjustment disorder with anxiety (American Psychiatric Association 1994), where the stressor is a serious medical illness. But because most of these patients are chronically ill and have been in distress for many years, they fall between the diagnostic cracks of entities in DSM-IV, somewhere between anxiety disorders and somatoform disorders. (In DSM-III-R [American Psychiatric Association 1987], it was asserted that a coexisting disease may very well be present and that the person readily acknowledges that he or she may be exaggerating the extent of the feared disease.) According to Barsky and associates (1990), among general medical outpatients, functional somatic symptoms are actually more common after recovery from a serious medical illness than they are at other times, and illness has been found to precipitate anxiety that Barsky et al. characterized as hypochondriacal.

Bodily complaints often are the initial symptoms in people with schizo-phrenia, presenting when they are in their late teens; these symptoms are the earliest flickers of somatic delusions that become fixed and intractable as the disease progresses. I saw my share of these young individuals in the 7 years that I was a consultant to a plastic surgery service (Druss et al. 1971). These people describe their symptoms in an odd way, with frequent oblique references to their appearance and physical development, beyond the ex-pected concerns of any normal adolescent. At the other end of the chrono-logical spectrum are the depressions of late middle age and old age, which may arise in formerly sanguine individuals; they too present with morbid bodily worries, often centered on the gastrointestinal tract. They are overtly depressed and usually do not present a diagnostic problem. In milder ver-sions, "masked depressions" hiding behind somatic complaints are a diag-nostic challenge for internists as well as mental health professionals (Derogatis and Wise 1989).

There is a vast literature on hypochondriasis. This literature delineates the unpopularity of these patients with the physicians caring for them (who may use such terms as "crock," often with the implication of malingerer), the phenomenon of secondary gain and motivation for compensation, the futility of reassurance, the intractability of hypochondriasis, and the often-described paradoxical aggravation of hypochondriasis with medical and surgical intervention. These views, shared by the medical community, often lessen the opportunity for good medical care for these patients. An addi-tional burden they may bear is the insight that their fears are exaggerated, leading to shame, concerns about cowardice, and lowered self-esteem.

I have chosen a few references that I hope will shed light on why some chronically ill people become overconcerned, offer a very tentative hypoth-esis of my own based on clinical experience, and then describe some of the ways that hypochondriasis can be ameliorated and mitigated, even if not cured.

Review of the Literature

Fenichel (1945) devoted a section of his book *The Psychoanalytic Theory of Neurosis* to the classical psychoanalytic view of hypochondriasis. He felt that hypochondriasis was rarely an isolated neurosis, but more frequently was a factor complicating some other psychopathological condition, and that it involved a withdrawal of "psychic energy" from the outside world to the bodily organs. He felt that the psychoanalytic process often reveals that the hypochondriacal concerns are displacements from childhood anxiety about mutilation and that certain unnamed childhood experiences have transformed that anxiety into a "sickness phobia." Fenichel also implied that a lack of "adequate discharge" of emotions may actually heighten the tension in certain bodily organs, causing an increased sense of awareness—not a big leap from Freud's early theory of actual neurosis (1896). To the best of my knowledge, Freud, so interested in the mind-body interface throughout his life, has but one tiny reference to hypochondriasis per se in his entire oeuvres.

Thomas Szasz, in his brilliant book *Pain and Pleasure* (1957), discussed hypochondriasis from a different point of view. He described normal everyday orientation to the body as largely neutral—the way we wash and dress in the morning, knowing what we are doing but without special attention or interest. He felt that some people are unduly "interested" in the functioning of their body and have curiosity about whether it functions properly. He described these people with an increased interest as "hypochondriacs" and suggested that bodily interests tend to overshadow all others. The individual becomes totally focused on his or her own body. He or she begins to perceive sensations that call attention to bodily parts: look here, touch there. Pain and itching are such examples. Parts of the body may therefore torment the hypochondriacal person, much as delusional figures seem to torment paranoid persons. The individual must continually respond to the demands for attention from that potentially threatening internal body part. Szasz thus bridges the gap between the psychoanalytic view of the defense mechanism of displacement and a cognitive view of selective attention.

The cognitive etiology of hypochondriasis is discussed by Barsky and associates (1988). They see hypochondriasis as an "amplification disorder" in which normal bodily sensations and the somatic components of affect are amplified into something harmful, and the individual believes himself or herself to be seriously ill. For example, once a person suspects he or she has emphysema, normal exertional dyspnea supports and consolidates this erroneous supposition. These authors offered many research studies suggesting that people with hypochondriasis exhibit lower pain thresholds. They also cited other studies that demonstrate that hypochondriacal people misattribute normal bodily sensations to symptoms of illness rather than to fatigue, dietary indiscretion, or overwork. They cited additional data suggesting that medically ill people may develop transient hypochondriasis because the illness itself can amplify somatosensory stimuli.

Hypochondriasis has also been characterized as a behavioral disorder in which the "sick role" was learned early in life (Kolb 1968). It is more frequently manifested by people who have shown a previous tendency to gain attention or evade responsibilities of life through illness. Kolb further felt that parents, themselves worried over health matters, would be a major source of this tendency. Fearful parents produce fearful offspring and impart the view that our world is a germ-laden, plague-ridden field of land mines.

Some hypochondriasis is iatrogenic. Physicians may scare their patients. More and more, the fear of malpractice leads to value "honesty" about risks and side effects. Informed consent is a mixed blessing, with more emphasis given to the consent and less to necessary careful informing. But a physician can also say too much. Any patient who would consult the *Physicians' Desk Reference* with its endless list of side effects would be reluctant to take any medication whatsoever. At times, the hypochondriacal patient, worrying over every symptom, engenders counterhostility in the physician. These are not the busy practitioner's favorite patients because they require more time and repetition. But a recent study by Starcevic (1991) showed that explanation, when properly done and with the right patient, is enormously ameliorative of hypochondriacal anxieties, whether they be related to the condition, the diagnostic procedures, or the proposed medical or surgical treatment.

By far the most interesting biological studies of hypochondriasis are being conducted by Fallon and his associates (1991, 1993a, 1993b). They noted that at times it was difficult to distinguish hypochondriasis from obsessive-compulsive disorder (OCD). Much like the patient with OCD, the hypochondriacal patient is "obsessed with intrusive thoughts and plagued with the tyranny of uncertainty" (Fallon et al. 1993b, p. 374). And like the OCD patient, the person with hypochondriasis "has compulsive behaviors: bodily 'checking' or repeatedly seeking reassurances from a relative or physician" (Fallon et al. 1993b, p. 375). Fallon et al. reported that fluoxetine, useful in the treatment of OCD, is also helpful in the treatment of hypochondriasis. It is interesting to note that doses of 60 mg or more of fluoxetine were effective, whereas doses of 20–40 mg were not. Fluoxetine, a serotonin reuptake inhibitor, has been shown to be a useful agent in the treatment of major depression, but the lower doses often effective in depression are insufficient to treat OCD or hypochondriasis.

Another pharmacological approach may be necessary in individuals who are chronic worriers. They have what is called "generalized" or "free-floating" anxiety, especially in anticipation of fearful events. The discovery of benzodiazepine receptor sites lends credence to a lifelong deficiency state responsible for a lifelong propensity to anticipatory anxiety. These patients often respond to treatment with benzodiazepines (Arana and Hyman 1991; Derogatis and Wise 1989).

Case Reports

Case 1

Mr. M. was a 50-year-old man who was referred by his internist. About 2 months previously, at a routine examination, he had been found to have "mild clinical diabetes" and had become extremely anxious, almost to the point of panic, ever since. He was totally preoccupied with thoughts of the dire consequences of diabetes, especially the circulatory sequelae, and was secretly feeling his foot and ankle pulses throughout the day.

He told me that he had been concerned about his health as far back as he could remember, despite a lifetime of excellent health, and the diagnosis of diabetes was the coup de grace, transforming a worry into a reality. For example, he recalled that during his teens he would read in the newspaper the accounts of the number of cases of poliomyelitis each summer and breathe a sigh of relief each Labor Day. At the movies, when the annual March of Dimes fund-raiser was in progress, he would often have to absent himself when young people in crutches were depicted.

Other than this particular symptom pattern, he presented himself as a rather cautious but successful businessman, with a happy, fulfilling marital and social life. He had never been "depressed or pessimistic" until his internist sounded this "knell of doom."

I suggested that psychodynamic psychotherapy might be the treatment of choice because his symptoms appeared to be deeply rooted in forgotten past events. He readily agreed to psychotherapy, and the acute nature of his apprehensions faded rather quickly. It was in the course of his self-scrutiny that he chanced to speak to his elder brother about their early childhood. He learned (but did not recall) that his father's mother had lived two flights above them in New York, and that she had had diabetes. One nightmarish memory vividly emerged. He recalled being cared for by and left alone with this grandmother. At one point, she had removed a heavy orthopedic shoe and revealed a foot with all the toes amputated. He had a memory of her stocking tucked in at the end. His grandmother died when he was 3, so this encounter occurred before then.

Case 2

Dr. N., a physician, entered psychodynamic psychotherapy at age 39 after a long series of unsatisfactory relationships with men. She was able to put aside her attraction to cruel, unfaithful men and by the end of treatment some 7 years later was happily married. A related but secondary issue that slowly emerged during the therapy was her frequent use of medical consultations for a wide variety of minor concerns well beyond what she referred to as "second-year medical student syndrome." She saw allergists, dermatologists, gynecologists, and so on, always with much worry and apprehension. She felt that she had identified with her mother, who was a fearful woman, especially about illness and injury, and who initiated the patient's career of doctor shopping. It was clear that she entered medicine with the hope of mastering her fear of physical illness.

She had avoided athletics most of her life, but her husband, a fine athlete, persuaded her to join him in his avocation of running. She reluctantly agreed and, to her surprise and pleasure, enjoyed it immensely. She felt physically well for the first time, and the experience of running appeared to address the issue of passivity that was the major focus of her therapy. She ran daily and was feeling as robust as I had seen her when, on a weekend run, an impatient jogger accidentally tripped her and she fell, twisting her knee painfully.

She was found to have no fracture but was given a rigid knee brace and running was interdicted for 6 months. Her mood plummeted, and apprehensions that she had an infection or even osteogenic sarcoma of the tibia began to preoccupy her. It was in this state, which lasted during her 5–6 months of incapacity, that we looked at hitherto untouched history.

She had been told that during her first year of life she had contracted a variant of Guillain-Barré syndrome, which led to weakness in her legs and delayed her walking. She never needed hospitalization but required home nursing and painful physical therapy. This illness had a devastating effect on her mother. Dr. N. felt that this initiated her mother's preoccupation with the patient's health and physical welfare and the myth of Dr. N.'s helplessness and passivity. Even after the running injury healed totally, she returned to her "hypochondriacal" ways, and the insights gained during this period did not alter them. To the best of my knowledge, this injury, perceived as punishment for physical assertion, ended her brief athletic career.

Case 3

The third patient was an 11-year-old girl with an incompletely closed soft palate who had become terrified at the prospect of the simple procedure that would approximate the opening. Until about 2 months previously, she had welcomed the surgery because although she was a beautiful, angelic child, her voice had a guttural, adenoidal tone, and she had begun to be mimicked and teased by classmates. Such surgery is not done until the face is fully mature, or it would have been proposed much earlier.

The open palate had led to some problems with nursing and early feeding, which worried her overprotective mother. The girl was a thin child, but never undernourished, and she had no fear of injections, dental work, or doctors.

I began twice-a-week psychodynamic psychotherapy, which she took to readily. She couldn't explain her new fear of the surgery but had vivid dreams of spears, arrows, and pencils puncturing her mouth and her abdomen. She had considerable unconscious confusion about her bodily orifices. She was angry at her mother's infantilization of her; she was dressed like a 7- or 8-year-old even though she had just begun junior high school.

As the treatment proceeded, she discussed her father more. He was strict with bedtime, homework, and chores and treated her and her mother and younger brother harshly. She then described her public spankings. He would be seated in the living room with her head face down in his lap. He would lift her skirt, exposing her panties, and slap her repeatedly on the backside. She felt humiliated and at times would be sick to her stomach. I called both parents into my office for a special session. Looking directly at the father I said, "Your daughter is getting too old to spank," and the spankings stopped.

During the course of treatment, her apprehensions about the surgery began to diminish, and she had dreams of being a movie star or a television personality. She underwent the surgery without a hitch, and I saw her once more, a month later. The change in her appearance was dramatic. She wore stockings and age-appropriate clothing and was less open and chatty. She said school was more important than treatment now, and it was time to stop. She thanked me for all my help, but in the distant and rather aloof manner of an adolescent. Her mother contacted me a year later to say that she was a social butterfly and that all was well.

Discussion

As I said, these cases taken from my practice are typical. A review of my patient records suggested to me that many individuals with hypochondriasis were traumatized during the first 2 years of life. Specifically, they often were seriously ill themselves or were exposed to an ill person in their immediate family. Therefore, a generalized anxiety state leads quite directly to a fear of illness and an anamnestic response when illness occurs, instead of taking off in a variety of other possible directions.

The kind of traumatic experiences I am referring to might include burns and scalds, the latter leaving no physical scar. It would include surgery for various conditions, including the one-time obligatory tonsillectomy. Other examples might be various orthopedic devices with leg-twisting braces and boots and various procedures for correcting congenital defects. The disease or defect itself is not important. What is important is the sense of helplessness and victimization that one imagines an infant might feel by the poking, the painful examinations, and frequent invasions by others. These serve to violate an infant's body boundaries and developing sense of body image. And, because the child is young, there is insufficient ego to process these experiences, and he or she responds only with an autonomic discharge of helplessness and rage. If the child is in addition born with a lower pain threshold, his or her suffering would be further magnified.

Exposure to a chronically ill relative may operate in a similar way. The child is horrified. How did it happen? Can it happen to me? Is he or she in pain? Chronic exposure in childhood to handicapped people or people with painful illnesses may be overwhelming and traumatic.

The theory that those who get a disease or who view it in others at an early age are at risk for hypochondriasis is merely a hypothesis. If these traumas occur during the first year or two of life, they will not be easily remembered. But no treatment of a hypochondriacal patient is complete without a careful inquiry into the early medical health of the patient and his or her childhood caretakers. How this trauma and the accompanying anxiety are altered and woven into the developmental conflicts of any individual patient's psychological life is part of the work entailed in understanding these patients.

Case 1 involved a man who was in good health all his life. The initial traumas involved contact with his deformed grandmother, which left him worried about his health all his life, fearing physical injury and deformity. It left him vulnerable to the diabetes when it was diagnosed later in life. But it was not the possibility of repeated episodes of diabetic acidosis, blindness, kidney disease, etc., that concerned him; it was quite specifically the possibility of becoming crippled in his legs like his grandmother. Fear of polio as an adolescent was another example of this rather specific concern. Hypochondriasis may not necessarily be vague or fluctuating, but rather specific in nature.

Case 2 has a vaguer quality. The woman's fears were more generalized, and when she developed a knee injury her concerns were less specific, ranging from infection to cancer. My formulation of this case is that the original trauma, her Guillain-Barré syndrome, is a vague fluctuating disorder with many symptoms, including paralysis, bladder and bowel problems, and perhaps even difficulty breathing. Also, the original condition occurred when she was very young, before she had the same powers of observation and intellectual organization as the patient in Case 1.

The third patient, the preteenager, is especially interesting, and her situation was less common. There were two traumas: the open palate leading to feeding problems in her infancy centering around interaction with her mother was the first; a series of spankings from her father with her face in his lap was the second. The fact that she was high functioning, open, and sociable prevented a phobia from becoming a more serious mental disorder. Her parents' cooperation, her own strong motivation to be normal and accepted, and her psychological aptitude aided in the treatment process.

Treatment

The cornerstone of good treatment for these patients is that they be in the hands of an empathic primary internist, surgeon, orthopedist, etc., who is not put off by many questions and doubts and is clear in his or her explanations. Some patients want to be partners of the physician and treated as equals; some wish for a benign father who says, "Leave all the worrying to me"; and some want the satisfaction of a meticulous workup. What stands for reassurance differs for each patient. But the idea that reassurance is of no use at all in hypochondriasis is a myth that needs to be dispelled (Starcevic 1991). It just has to be the right kind of reassurance, suited to the patient and based on a good doctor-patient relationship.

Psychiatrists should be knowledgeable about the patient's particular disease, to aid in assessing the situation, and should reinforce any reassurance in cases that warrant it. The psychiatrist should also ensure that patients are satisfied with their medical care and, if they are not, explore why patients are not getting what they need.

I have described many causes of hypochondriasis, and all must be addressed. Because I am hypothesizing that very early illness or exposure to illness of others in childhood may put one at risk for later hypochondriasis, psychodynamic psychotherapy can focus on the recovery of repressed memories. Here the process bears similarities to psychiatry at the battlefield for what was called "shell shock" in World War I and "combat fatigue" in World War II. The treatment at that time involved abreaction of the trauma, at times with thiopental sodium. The medical and psychiatric disorders were treated in the same setting, and often the latter would respond quickly and dramatically. Pride in the unit, appeals to bravery, brief rest, and reassurance all played their part. But such brisk results should not regularly be expected in hypochondriasis because the causative events usually have occurred before the age of awareness. One encourages inquiry from parents and siblings and any other jolts to the memory. If necessary, there will be plenty of time later for more traditional free association, transference interpretation, and working through.

Many patients do well with cognitive therapy (Barsky et al. 1988). The therapeutic alliance stands in opposition to pessimism, regression, and the focus on limitations and emphasizes the coping mechanisms and strengths the patient already possesses. Specific training in ridding the mind of negative thinking and fear is a proven technique for some patients.

Finally, for the few days before any feared procedure or examination for recurrence, or the wait for the result of a biopsy, no insight will help. Keeping busy, diverted, and distracted is useful advice. And when even that fails, the patient may require judicious use of benzodiazepines for 3–5 days, and it would be cruel to withhold them. Calls and extra sessions should not be encouraged but may be necessary.

Ultimately, appeals to the patient's courage and endurance will have to grapple with the dread; the patient, like the soldier on the eve of combat, is on his or her own.

References

American Psychiatric Association: Diagnostic and Statistical Manual of Mental Disorders, 3rd Edition, Revised. Washington, DC, American Psychiatric Association, 1987

American Psychiatric Association: Diagnostic and Statistical Manual of Mental Disorders, 4th Edition. Washington, DC, American Psychiatric Association, 1994

Arana GW, Hyman SE: Handbook of Psychiatric Drug Therapy, 2nd Edition. Boston, MA, Little, Brown, 1991

Barsky AJ, Geringer E, Wool CA: A cognitive-educational treatment for hypochondriasis. Gen Hosp Psychiatry 10:322–327, 1988

Barsky A, Wyshak G, Klerman G: Transient hypochondriasis. Arch Gen Psychiatry 47:746–752, 1990

Derogatis LR, Wise TN: Anxiety and Depressive Disorders in the Medical Patient. Washington, DC, American Psychiatric Press, 1989

Druss RG, Symonds FC, Crikelair GF: The problem of somatic delusions in patients seeking cosmetic surgery. Journal of Plastic and Reconstructive Surgery 48:246–250, 1971

Fallon B, Javitch J, Hollander E, et al: Hypochondriasis and obsessive compulsive disorder: overlaps in diagnosis and treatment. J Clin Psychiatry 52:457–460, 1991

Fallon BA, Rasmussen SA, Liebowitz MP: Hypochondriasis, in Obsessive-Compulsive–Related Disorders. Edited by Hollander E. Washington, DC, American Psychiatric Press, 1993a, pp 71–92

Fallon B, Klein B, Liebowitz M: Hypochondriasis: treatment strategies. Psychiatric Annals 23:374–381, 1993b

Fenichel O: The Psychoanalytic Theory of Neurosis. New York, WW Norton, 1945

Freud S: Further remarks on the neuropsychoses of defence (1896), in the Standard Edition of the Complete Psychological Works of Sigmund Freud, Vol 3. Translated and edited by Strachey J. London, Hogarth Press, 1962, pp 159–185

Kolb L: Modern Clinical Psychiatry, 7th Edition. New York, WB Saunders, 1968

Physicians' Desk Reference, 48th Edition. Montvale, NJ, Medical Economics Data, 1994

Starcevic V: Reassurance and treatment of hypochondriasis. Gen Hosp Psychiatry 13:122–127, 1991

Szasz T: Pain and Pleasure. New York, Basic Books, 1957

3

Pathological Denial

Denial is a common response to illness. It is a defense mechanism that may take a variety of forms, including ignoring warning symptoms, postponing medical evaluation, or refusing recommended treatment (Hackett and Cassem 1974; Schmale 1979). In this chapter, I begin by describing two dramatic examples of denial of illness. The cases are unusual and noteworthy because of the severe and debilitating nature of the symptoms tolerated by these individuals over many years before they sought help. I speculate on reasons for their initial avoidance of medical attention and for their subsequent negative reaction to medical treatment and offer a hypothesis of how these two common behaviors are linked psychodynamically. The hope is that an in-depth examination of these two extreme cases will provide a place to begin a discussion of denial of illness. Pathological denial is also commonly seen in everyday life. There are times when it has profound consequences.

Portions of this chapter are adapted by permission of the publisher from Douglas CJ, Druss RG: "Denial of Illness: A Reappraisal." *General Hospital Psychiatry* 9:53–57, 1987. Copyright 1987 by Elsevier Science Publishing Co., Inc.

Case Reports

Case 1

Ms. A., a 43-year-old, divorced woman, presented to our emergency room complaining of severe facial pain. She was wearing a surgical mask over her face. When the mask was removed, a disfigured face was revealed. Her nose was totally destroyed, her lips were mutilated, and there were numerous badly scarred, necrotic, and infected areas on her eyelids and the periphery of her face. Her eyes, which she could hardly close, teared continuously. The overall effect was a horror-show fixed grin. The rest of her physical and neurological examination was otherwise unremarkable.

The hospital chart indicated that she had visited the emergency room 11 years earlier because of a small, painless "scab" on her nose. An appointment was made for her in the dermatology clinic the next day. She did not keep the appointment nor did she answer follow-up letters from the hospital. In fact, she did not return to seek medical attention for over a decade.

As the lesion grew, leaving her more disfigured, she progressively isolated herself in her apartment. On the few occasions when she did venture out, she wore the face mask and traveled across rooftops to avoid being seen. Only when the lesion invaded bone and the pain became intolerable did she finally return to the emergency room and accept hospitalization.

A biopsy of her skin lesions on admission showed a noncaseating granulomatous disease, which proved to be tertiary syphilis. Serologic tests for syphilis (ART and FTA-ABS) were reactive, and she received a course of intramuscular penicillin. A lumbar puncture was not performed. After some hesitation, she agreed to undergo plastic surgery to reconstruct her nose.

In a series of staged procedures, a flap of skin from the arm and bone from the iliac crest were successfully refashioned into a nose. Several months later, however, the nasal tip became infected, resulting in gradual reabsorption of the shape of the nose. Ms. A. admitted that despite warnings from her doctors, she had continued to wear the face mask after the surgery.

A year later, reconstructive surgery was again attempted, using a Silastic implant. However, a wound infection mysteriously developed postoperatively, and the implant was removed. Four months after this, a flap of skin from the other arm was successfully grafted to reform the nose but again became quickly ulcerated. By this time, the surgical team became suspicious that the lesions had been self-inflicted. Psychiatric consultation was requested.

The consultant found Ms. A. to be aloof, distant, and suspicious. She was only mildly depressed, denied neurovegetative signs of depression, and showed no clear signs of psychosis or organic impairment. She volunteered little information about herself and was reluctant to discuss her feelings concerning the illness and surgery. She said only that she felt "hurt" about having syphilis, unjustly afflicted with a disease she associated with promiscuity.

The eldest of four children born to working-class parents from the rural South, Ms. A. had been obliged to quit school after the 10th grade to help support the family. She had led a quiet, isolated existence most of her life except for a brief, strained marriage when she was in her early 20s that had ended in divorce. She moved in with her mother after the divorce, "lost interest" in men, and occupied herself doing domestic work for neighbors in her building. After she developed the "spot" on her nose, she became a virtual recluse. She worried that she might have cancer but was intensely afraid of hospitals and doctors, whom she had always regarded as "mean." She traced these fears to a traumatic series of examinations and injections that she received when she was 4 years old. Her fear of physicians intensified at age 13 when her father died unexpectedly during surgery for head trauma sustained in a mugging.

Ms. A. insisted that she was disappointed that the two previous reconstructive procedures had failed and wished only to "pick my life up again and go back to work." However, the social worker to whom she had been referred during her first admission noted that she was having trouble keeping appointments and "continued to have a difficult time establishing even a minimal relationship with anyone." With support from the consultant and the social worker, Ms. A. was able to make some small strides toward becoming more independent, such as shopping alone for groceries and obtaining a high school equivalency degree. The nasal ulcers healed, and this time there was no recurrence of infection. Ten years later, however, the patient continued to lead a socially marginal life and had not returned to work.

Case 2

Ms. R., a 51-year-old, single tax specialist, was brought to the emergency room by her sisters because she had been acting "dazed and confused." In retrospect, the family realized that for about a year, she had seemed unusually anxious, distracted, and forgetful. She became more withdrawn, ignored housework, and stopped opening her mail. For the first time in her 27 years with her company, she began to have trouble functioning at work. A supervisor had recently warned her that if she did not improve her performance she would be fired. Nevertheless, she had adamantly opposed her family's efforts to get her to a doctor until she became frankly disoriented.

The examining physician discovered a loud flow murmur and an enlarged uterus, which he described as being "the size of a 7-month pregnancy." Routine laboratory studies were notable for a hemoglobin of 4.5 mmol/L. On closer questioning, it was learned that 12 years earlier Ms. R. had developed menorrhagia and was told by her gynecologist that she had fibroids. She refused surgery because she was terrified of hospitals and physicians. She preferred to suffer heavy vaginal bleeding (requiring up to 20 sanitary napkins daily) rather than return to see the gynecologist. She seemed unconcerned about her gradually increasing abdominal girth. In fact, family members recalled that she often patted her expanding belly affectionately and joked about the "baby in there."

Over her strenuous objections, she was admitted to the hospital. After receiving several blood transfusions, she underwent an emergency hysterectomy without complications. Her confusion, which was attributed to severe anemia and cerebral hypoxia, cleared, and she was discharged 8 days later. However, several weeks after her discharge, she began to look sad and worried. She became increasingly fearful and suspicious, kept the lights burning at night, and accused her sisters of talking behind her back. Vegetative symptoms included decreased appetite, a 15-pound weight loss, early and terminal insomnia, listlessness, and an inability to concentrate. She was unable to return to work. After 4 months in this state, she very reluctantly allowed her family to bring her back to the emergency room, and she was admitted to our psychiatric service.

Ms. R. was frail and apprehensive. She wore her hair in two long braids, which gave her an almost girlish appearance. Extremely vigilant and guarded, she offered only brief, vague answers to questions. Although she had mild deficits in attention, concentration, and short-term memory, an extensive workup did not reveal any organic cause for her psychiatric syndrome. She admitted that she had felt frightened of doctors since she was 8 years old, when a needle broke off in her arm during a routine vaccination. She had postponed the hysterectomy because she was firmly convinced she would die on the operating table. Yet she now worried that she had waited too long to have the fibroids removed, allowing them to "turn into cancer." She added somewhat blandly that after the operation, she had also "suddenly realized" that she had lost the potential to have children, which she regretted.

She was the youngest of eight children in an impoverished family from Florida. Her father had abandoned the family before she was born. She joined her accounting firm after graduating from college and had worked there ever since. Although well liked by co-workers, she had few close friends and had always been shy and taciturn. She had received several marriage proposals when she was younger but had turned them down because "it was never the right man." She lived alone and had little social contact with people other than her immediate family.

She was believed to have a major depression with psychotic features and pseudodementia and a schizoid character structure. Depressive symptoms and cognitive deficits responded over 1 month to a combination of desipramine and haloperidol. However, at the time of discharge, Ms. R. remained isolated, cautious, and suspicious. A year later, she still had not returned to work.

Discussion

These cases raise two major issues. First, why did these women postpone medical care for so long? Second, why, after successful medical treatment, did their functioning continue to deteriorate rather than improve? These two patients, both very disturbed, manifest an extreme form of denial and neglect of illness. But denial almost as severe in otherwise "normal" individuals has been described in the literature. Hackett and Cassem (1975) cited cases of men who had chest pains and who, in the midst of a developing heart attack, did vigorous push-ups or climbed flights of stairs to convince themselves that what they were experiencing was not a myocardial infarct. Katz et al. (1970) reported a study of 30 women who had discovered a breast lump. Denial and rationalization were serious enough in all 30 to delay their getting proper medical attention.

More recently, Strauss et al. (1990) indicated how frequently denial of physical illness occurs in a consultation-liaison psychiatry setting. These authors presented eight typical but different kinds of cases. They concluded that the condition is so common that DSM-IV should include a subtype of adjustment disorder called "with maladaptive denial of physical disorder." In one case, they specifically addressed the issue of differential diagnosis from psychosis: "In a psychotic disorder, the individual not only has impaired reality testing but creates a new reality. In maladaptive denial of physical illness, the individual is insisting on the old reality rather than creating a new reality. Therefore a diagnosis of psychosis is not appropriate" (p. 1171).

A number of explanations could be offered for the tenacity with which the women I've discussed resisted medical attention. First, both were raised in families in which skepticism about physicians was widely endorsed and eschewal of medical treatment was culturally sanctioned (Becker and Maiman 1975). Second, anxiety-provoking medical experiences in childhood left them both with a phobic attitude toward medical care. Subsequent contact with physicians would be expected to reawaken strong fears of bodily injury. Third, the symbolic meaning of illness can often arouse in the patient more powerful fear than the illness itself. For the patients I have described, the conditions directly threatened highly valued body parts (facial appearance) and bodily functions (reproduction) (Bernstein 1976). Anxiety about mutilation might well have been strong enough to supersede the more rational fear of cancer evoked by their disease. Fourth, certain personality traits that these women shared probably accounted in part for their retreat in the face of illness. Both had schizoid character structures and would be expected to respond to the stress of illness by withdrawal and intensification of denial (Mumford 1977). These factors, alone or in some combination, seem to explain the powerful denial of illness that allowed their conditions to proceed to such advanced stages.

The more difficult, but perhaps more interesting, question I must still address is why, after overcoming their fear of doctors and undergoing appropriate treatment for their illnesses, these women seemed to deteriorate further or to undermine their treatment rather than regain their premorbid level of functioning. It was strongly suspected that Ms. A. sabotaged efforts to reconstruct her nose. The reasons for this were never clear. Successful treatment of her depression did not enable her to return to a job that had previously been her major source of gratification. These developments are not adequately accounted for by the factors I outlined earlier, and other explanations must be sought. Because the patients provided little information about their inner experience of the illness and treatment, the interpretations I offer are admittedly somewhat speculative. A brief review of several analogous cases previously reported in the literature may clarify this issue.

Lettin (1964) described the unusual story of a 26-year-old woman who was advised to wear a plaster cast temporarily for back pain after a fall.

When her physician recommended some time later that the cast be removed or replaced by a less constricting corset, she left treatment. It was subsequently learned that she had continued to wear the same cast unchanged for 12 years, until abdominal pain forced her to return to the hospital. The cast had caused severe lumbar scoliosis and back rigidity. The author hypothesized that the patient had developed a psychological dependence on the plaster jacket: "The complete incapacity and the imploring letters which followed the removal of the plaster could be compared to withdrawal symptoms of the drug addict" (p. 795).

Certain morbidly obese individuals have been reported to become severely depressed or even psychotic after dieting and may regain the lost weight rapidly (Robinson and Winnik 1973). Crisp and Stonehill (1970) reported the case of a massively obese 24-year-old woman who, despite developing complications of diabetes, menorrhagia, and respiratory difficulty, refused treatment of her obesity for 12 years, until her doctor insisted that her life was in jeopardy. She reluctantly agreed to be admitted for a reducing diet and, over the course of a year, lost 85 pounds. However, she became severely depressed after discharge and was rehospitalized several months later after a serious suicide attempt. She rapidly returned to her obese state but remained profoundly depressed. A year later, she killed herself.

These cases might be likened to those of criminals who are paroled only to repeat the same offense for which they were originally jailed. Such recidivism has been attributed by Clemmer (1950) in part to a wish to return to the prison environment to which criminals have become so acculturated that they are unprepared for an extramural life.

The common denominator in these cases is that illness became a necessary condition for patients' sense of security and well-being. I do not believe this is explained by secondary gain derived from assuming the "sick role," as postulated by Gallagher (1978). In fact, my patients tended to ignore symptoms and vigorously avoided medical attention. Rather, I feel, for certain patients, illness may come to serve important organizing and integrating functions. First, illness, like prison, may provide a kind of sheltered environment that allows avoidance of conflictual situations and protects areas of dysfunction. For example, the facial disfigurement of Ms. A. and the heavy vaginal bleeding of Ms. R. justified a retreat from social interaction and shielded them from the demands of interpersonal relationships. Just as a muscle atrophies through lack of normal exercise, it may be that the ability to resume the "healthy role" in the outside world is gradually lost.

Second, the failure of these patients to cooperate with or benefit from treatment might be regarded as a variant of the negative therapeutic reaction. The concept of negative therapeutic reaction was first suggested by Freud in 1923. The definition was clarified by Moore and Fine (1990, p. 125) as "a seemingly paradoxical response where there is a worsening of a patient's condition after an effective therapeutic management." Kernberg (1988) offered two elaborations. The less pathological motivation is derived from an unconscious sense of guilt in depressive-masochistic patients and is seen in patients unable to tolerate any success or improvement. A second, more serious motivation is the sadistic need to defeat the helper and is seen in self-destructive primitive individuals. For these patients, the failure to benefit from treatment may have gratified unconscious wishes to defeat or triumph over their doctors.

Third, although illness can be experienced initially by such patients as an invading enemy, over time it may become a kind of familiar old friend and eventually a part of the self. Bodily changes associated with the disease become integrated into patients' views of themselves and into their body schema. A similar process has been described in patients who undergo surgical alterations in body structure in adult life. I reported (1973) that women who undergo breast augmentation may experience profound changes not only in body image but also in the ego or self. According to Castelnuovo-Tedesco (1973), significant characterological changes have also been described in patients who receive kidney transplants. He noted that the kidney recipient would frequently take on personality characteristics of the donor. The donor was a close relative, most often a sibling or a parent, and therefore known to the patient. For example, a timid patient might feel more outgoing after receiving a transplant from a more assertive older brother. Viederman's (1971) interesting work with patients who received kidney transplants indicated that patients often "accept" or "reject" the organ depending on their psychological as well as physiological relationship with the donor.

The example of my patients suggests that if illness is permitted to last long enough, it too may become incorporated into the view of the self and lead to basic ego modifications. This construction of the self is forged slowly and cannot be easily dislodged. I believe this is particularly true for patients like the women I have described whose rigid character structure and limited repertoire of coping skills make adaptation to change more difficult. Treatment of their illness would be paradoxically experienced as a threat to the basic sense of intactness and integrity of the self, as discussed by Lichtenberg (1975). Maintaining a stable and consistent view of the self for such individuals ultimately becomes more important than the preservation or restoration of their physical health. To use Lettin's (1964) case as an analogy, the plaster cast eventually became an indispensable "exoskeleton" without which his patient felt utterly disabled and unable to function.

I further believe, for certain patients, illness and the bodily changes it causes may verify premorbid views of the self as ugly, evil, or bad. Medical interventions, not surprisingly, would be resisted because the "improvements" in appearance afforded by treatment would no longer conform to these internalized, fixed, and distorted views of the self. In other words, the "denial of illness" and subsequent "refusal to get well" may *both* derive from a need to maintain not simply a consistent view of the self, as suggested earlier, but a specific, long-standing, pathological view of the self. Thus, in addition to the various cultural and intrapsychic factors I have reviewed, one important determinant in patients' avoiding and then failing to benefit from medical treatment may be these early, defective self-images that are in some manner validated by their physical illness. Psychological interventions with these difficult patients would have to address these basic deficits in self-esteem if medical treatment is to be helpful.

Denial in Everyday Life

Pathological denial of a different but related nature can be seen in so many individuals that one can almost refer to a *denial in everyday life*. The psychopathology is less severe than I discussed earlier, but the consequences of it are no less dangerous. What can we say of the woman over 40 who doesn't have regular Pap smears of the cervix? Or of men and women over 40 who haven't had a routine physical examination in a decade? And of men and women of all ages who are practicing unsafe sex in the age of AIDS? All are using pathological denial regarding their health, with potentially serious consequences. (None of this is "creative risk taking," to be discussed in Chapter 6, "Healthy Denial.")

Some very common everyday activities illustrate these types of frequent and often dangerous behavior. The first is smoking. No public health problem has received such wide publicity, with such convincing evidence from the surgeon general on down, as has cigarette smoking. Smoking is now banned from airplanes and many public institutions like hospitals and libraries, and warnings are displayed even on the cigarette packages themselves. Why do some people continue to smoke? A study of 97 smokers and 95 nonsmokers, ranging in age from 15 to 65 years, was conducted by Lee (1989). She found strong evidence supporting denial of *risk* in the smokers: they believe that their own risk is less than that of the average smoker. Not surprisingly, this factor was more pronounced in younger smokers in her sample. Such denial of risk undermines the effectiveness of stop-smoking campaigns, Lee feels, and I agree.

My office is located near two prestigious, competitive, women's prep schools. I take my lunch at a diner nearby once or twice a month. The tables are filled with women of high school age, and I am usually the only non-smoker. Smoking is clearly a ritual that they share, all wanting to conform and participate in a grown-up activity. Group pressure and group acceptance are crucial at that age. Their school-girl chatter about dates, grades, and vacations has not once included the perfunctory disclaimer that most adult smokers would murmur about risk before they light up. I feel like standing on a table and shouting, "Stop!" but have prudently kept my tongue. Lee's study (1989) suggests that sadly my jeremiad would fall on deaf ears.

Another example is seat belts. To quote Weinstein et al. (1986, p. 285), "the argument for using automobile seat belts seems overwhelming. The risk of death or serious injury in automobile accidents is large; seat belts are effective; and the effort to use them is minimal." The public does not disagree, and Weinstein et al. quoted three studies to back up this appraisal. With such low costs and high benefits, seat belt use should be almost universal. Yet, according to the National Highway Safety Administration cited in their article, the actual figure is only 14%! The authors devised a program of interventions that involved a 1-week exposure to dashboard stickers and signs in the parking deck and cafeteria of a large corporation. They found that at one exit, seat belt use increased 31%. In their discussion of these results, the authors felt that the program worked simply by reminding people to perform the desired behavior and short-circuited the more deeply held denial mechanisms. The level of seat belt use was approaching 50% at the time of long-term follow-up. But they concluded that everyday human behavior contains many risk factors for health hazards, and there is still a great need for understanding why people will not adopt preventive measures more universally.

In this regard, Weinstein (1987) reported the results of a questionnaire he mailed to a random sample of 296 individuals to obtain comparative risk judgment for 32 different health hazards. Included was everything from heart attacks and cancer to developing a problem with alcohol or drugs. He found that excessive optimism regarding future risk was most correlated with the belief, usually incorrect, that if the problem has not yet appeared one is exempt from future risk. This belief played a surprisingly powerful role in the appraisal of potential health hazards and was the most important new finding of this large study. The seriousness of the hazard was not correlated with degree of denial. Clearly, it is not sufficient for the public to know the realities of major risk factors for any given disease. Weinstein concluded that people are quite ingenious in finding reasons for believing that their own risk is less than everybody else's.

Physicians are not immune from these pathological denial mechanisms. Spiro (1990), a gastroenterologist, presented case histories of six physicians with inflammatory bowel disease. Noteworthy in all the physicians' accounts of illness was the degree of denial, actually leading to serious complications in five of the six.

Breznitz (1983) went even further in describing the ubiquity of pathological denial. He used the term *denial of urgency* to describe individuals who are sophisticated enough to understand the importance of everyday behaviors like smoking, lack of exercise, and improper dietary habits as coronary risk factors but who continue to postpone corrective action in relation to them. None of the risk factors pose an immediate threat; so in these cases, he feels that rationalization appears to be the motivation for denial and a defense against anxiety.

Conclusion

Pathological denial is a complex phenomenon. It may actually be a cluster of entities, different but related:

First, it is clearly a defense mechanism against fear of illness or the discovery of future illness.

Second, in addition, there seems to be a need for the retention of the sick state and unwillingness to get medical attention as an organizing function in some disturbed individuals. We see not only preservation of the sick role and consequential secondary gain but also a persistence of a pathological view of the self and body image over time and a "refusal" to get well.

Third, pathological denial is also a cognitive problem in which risks are rationalized for a variety of reasons, including age, temperament, and belief system. Epidemiological data reveal the ubiquity of pathological denial as a public health problem.

In our offices, we must deal with a series of individual patients, not the public at large. We should be alert to all the possible causes of pathological denial to best be of help to those in our care.

References

Becker MH, Maiman LA: Sociobehavioral determinants of compliance with health and medical care recommendations. Medical Care 13:10–24, 1975

Bernstein N: Emotional Care of the Facially Burned and Disfigured. Boston, MA, Little, Brown, 1976, pp 23–40

Breznitz S (ed): The seven kinds of denial, in The Denial of Stress. New York, International Universities Press, 1983, pp 257–280

Castelnuovo-Tedesco P: Organ transplant, body image, psychosis. Psychoanal Q 42:349–363, 1973

Clemmer D: Observations on imprisonment as a source of criminality. Journal of Criminal Law and Criminology 41:311–319, 1950

Crisp AH, Stonehill E: Treatment of obesity with special reference to seven severely obese patients. J Psychosom Res 14:327–345, 1970

Druss RG: Changes in body image following augmentation breast surgery. International Journal of Psychoanalysis and Psychotherapy 2:248–256, 1973

Freud S: The ego and the id (1923), in The Standard Edition of the Complete Psychological Works of Sigmund Freud, Vol 19. Translated and edited by Strachey J. London, Hogarth Press, 1962, pp 3–66

Gallagher EB: Lines of reconstruction and extension in the Parsonian sociology of illness. Soc Sci Med 10:207–218, 1978

Hackett TP, Cassem N: Development of a quantitative rating scale to assess denial. J Psychosom Res 18:93–100, 1974

Hackett TP, Cassem N: Psychologic management of the myocardial infarction patient. Journal of Human Stress 1:25–38, 1975

Katz J, Wieller H, Gallagher EB, et al: Stress distress and ego defenses. Arch Gen Psychiatry 23:131–142, 1970

Kernberg O: Clinical dimensions of masochism, in Masochism: Current Psychoanalytic Perspectives. Edited by Glick R, Meyers D. New York, Analytic Press, 1988, pp 61–79

Lee C: Perceptions of immunity to disease in adult smokers. J Behav Med 12:267–277, 1989

Lettin AW: Addiction to plaster? Lancet 1:795, 1964

Lichtenberg J: The development of the sense of self. J Am Psychoanal Assoc 23:453–484, 1975

Moore B, Fine B (eds): Psychoanalytic Terms and Concepts. New Haven, CT, American Psychoanalytic Association and Yale University Press, 1990

Mumford E: The responses of patients to medical advice, in Understanding Human Behavior in Health and Illness. Edited by Simon RC, Pardes H. Baltimore, MD, Williams & Wilkins, 1977, pp 405–416

Robinson S, Winnik HZ: Severe psychotic disturbances following weight loss. Arch Gen Psychiatry 29:559–562, 1973

Schmale AH: Reactions to illness, in Liaison Psychiatry. Edited by Kimball C. Philadelphia, PA, WB Saunders, 1979, pp 321–330

Spiro H: Six physicians with inflammatory bowel disease. J Clin Gastroenterol 12:636–642, 1990

Strauss D, Spitzer R, Muskin P: Maladaptive denial of physical illness: a proposal for DSM-IV. Am J Psychiatry 147:1168–1172, 1990

Viederman M: Report presented to workshop on Psychic Consequences of Congenital Lack and Acquired Loss of Bodily Parts, American Psychoanalytic Association, New York, December 1971

Weinstein N: Unrealistic optimism about susceptibility to health problems: conclusions from a community-wide sample. J Behav Med 10:481–499, 1987

Weinstein N, Grub P, Vautier J: Increasing automobile seat belt use: an intervention emphasizing risk susceptibility. J Appl Psychol 71:285–290, 1986

4

Psychodynamic Psychotherapy With Patients With Serious Intercurrent Medical Illness

The treatment of patients with various intercurrent physical illnesses by psychodynamic psychotherapy has received little attention. I use the term *psychodynamic psychotherapy* as Gabbard (1992, 1994) does: a treatment modality that includes the exploration of unconscious conflicts and the reexperiencing of past relationships in the present in regular sessions with a clinician.

There are many reasons for this lack of attention. First, the classical psychosomatic model described in the pioneering studies by Karush and Daniels (1953), Margolin (1951), and Sperling (1967), in which the hope that intrapsychic conflict resolution and catharsis would ultimately *cure* the

Portions of this chapter are adapted by permission of the publisher from Druss RG: "Psychotherapy of Patients With Serious Intercurrent Medical Illness (Cancer)." *Journal of the American Academy of Psychoanalysis* 14:459–472, 1986.

medical illness, has not stood the test of time and is largely discredited. And, sadly, as a result, psychodynamic approaches to medically ill patients have often been thrown out with the bathwater.

At the same time, the consultation-liaison approach for acute illness has won wide appeal and shown proven efficacy. Here, somatic cure is not the therapeutic goal. Many psychiatrists in the liaison area have placed themselves on the medical "team" and consider this to be the most favorable locus for treating these patients (Strain and Grossman 1975). Supported by studies such as those conducted by Levitan and Kornfeld (1981) and Schindler et al. (1989), the cost-effectiveness of on-site psychiatric intervention has been clearly demonstrated. Also, supportive therapy as described by Finkel (1982), cognitive therapy by Haag (1984) and Greer et al. (1991), and group therapy by Fawzy et al. (1990, 1993) are useful techniques in the acute hospital setting. Education of nonpsychiatric physicians on the management of hospitalized patients is an indirect approach with similar goals and has been discussed by Garber (1990).

None of these methods address the day-to-day suffering of a patient when he or she leaves the hospital with a chronic, recurrent, or deteriorating disease that may linger on for years, not weeks. Only an office-based, ongoing therapy has something to offer this vast population functioning in society, often at a high level.

Many dynamically trained psychiatrists have been reluctant to make a long-term commitment to these patients. Some have wondered if a severe medical illness would prohibit an orderly exploration of an individual's intrapsychic life. The practical issues of their attending regular appointments have seemed insurmountable, and fitting someone with fluctuating health into one's daily schedule has discouraged others.

Finally, I reserve psychodynamic psychotherapy, and even psychoanalysis (Druss 1978), for a limited but significant group of medically ill patients. As a matter of fact, medical illness itself may motivate patients to seek the kind of life changes and reordering of priorities that only a psychodynamic approach can provide. (I discuss a wider range of treatment approaches in Chapter 5, "Treatment Philosophy.") Even in this age of statistical validation with control subjects and large sample sizes, there is still a place for an in-depth report of a single case with all its richness of detail.

Because I had previously treated cancer patients with psychodynamic psychotherapy, I decided that it would be the treatment of choice for the patient whose case history follows. The case narrative is used as a spring-board to formulate some general hypotheses about the psychology of ill-ness. Certain details have been omitted or altered to protect the anonymity of the patient.

Case Report

Ms. E. is a 35-year-old, married woman who entered treatment shortly after major surgery and chemotherapy for a retroperitoneal lymphoma. She de-scribed the surgical procedures, hospitalization, and chemotherapy as "un-pleasant" but was optimistic about the future, saying that her particular variant of the disease had a very high cure rate. She indicated total trust in her doctor's word. "What should I do with my life?" was the question she hoped to have answered by psychotherapy.

The patient herself was an attractive young woman. She dressed stylishly and lavishly. She was bright and quick and smiled readily. She in no way appeared sick and seemed almost too cheerful, too chatty, and too charming. I asked myself at that time, What is the prognosis of this illness? It was clear that she was denying the seriousness of her disorder. I was taken by her viva-cious manner, and we shared many interests and values. At any rate, the pa-tient felt that it was time for a thorough review of her life. We launched on a psychodynamic psychotherapy with a flexible frequency of 2–3 visits per week.

The early sessions were spent examining Ms. E.'s background and taking a thorough history. An only child, she was born in France. Her mother was artistic, strong-willed, and opinionated and was described as a physically un-demonstrative person. Her mother did not work but pursued her artistic interests at home. Her father was a lawyer—hard-working, dutiful, and rather bland. She recalled a special relationship with him during her early years but said he suffered a stroke that left him paralyzed and aphasic when she was 7 years old. After his stroke, she was sent to a boarding school: "My mother did not want me at home," she said. The patient did poorly in school despite high intelligence and was considered an underachiever. She was also regarded as rather aloof by classmates, but her attractiveness led both girls and boys to cluster around her, drawn by her bright eyes and fetching smile. The patient was good at athletics, perhaps something of a tomboy, artistic, and a good dancer. In her teenage years, she found special pleasure being the center of attention of male friends but grew up feeling that it was dangerous to give herself fully to any one person. She had never pursued a career.

She depicted a life with that special kind of pseudoindependence that one often sees in children sent off from home prematurely. She was competent, able, and "streetwise." She dated early and had shallow, superficial relationships with many men. Five years before her treatment, she married an older man, a talented architect with a fine reputation. He admired her, spoiled her, showered her with attention and gifts, and made all the decisions. She characterized him as competent, kind, and devoted to his work. They had one child, a son, 3 years old. The patient expressed much pleasure with her son, saying that he was a beautiful child; she liked to buy clothes for him and show him off. The affection for her son appeared to be genuine.

As the therapy progressed, the patient's comments were noted to be superficial, at times sarcastic, vaguely critical, and often a bit pouting. She had to be pressed to associate and reflect. She was action prone and ran rather than remembered. She tried to distract me with chitchat or to charm me with amusing anecdotes. She had little tolerance for my silence, and frequently there would be angry tears with threats to quit. The gentlest of clarifications, let alone interpretations, were reacted to as if they were criticisms of her very essence, and I offered them at my peril. We seemed to be getting nowhere, and I had doubts that we ever would. Although she was very bright, as the therapy progressed she appeared to have little psychological awareness and little motivation to change, and her defenses seemed unalterable.

It was many weeks into the therapy that she had her first two dreams. First dream: *I was mailing away a package of my old clothes.* Second dream: *The Smith family and I were enclosed in a cage. We were trying to escape by going over the bar. It was a restraining bar.* Her associations with the cage dealt with a concrete description of the cage itself and the arrangement of the various restraints. Although not apparent to her, it quickly became clear to me what she was describing, and I asked whether this was a dream of her hospital bed and the chemotherapy. She reacted strongly to this question and replied that she hated going to her internist for follow-up visits and found the experience frightening; it made her think about dying. She was convinced that she would not live to old age and then wondered whether the package of old clothes in her first dream was her, useless and to be cast off. The following sessions were filled with all the feelings previously repressed regarding her original surgery and chemotherapy: the indignities, the manhandling, the catheterizations, the pain that she had endured.

As the therapy proceeded, she began to talk at length about the relationship with her father. She uncovered early recollections on her own, and questions from me were no longer necessary. Angry feelings quickly surfaced; his stroke had, in effect, left her with neither parent. She hated the regimentation and loneliness of the boarding school. During the ensuing weeks, she vacillated between anger at her father's "desertion" and affection toward him for what he had given her in her very early years. The resolution she arrived at was that she *had* been Daddy's little princess early in life and had suffered an irreparable loss. This phase of treatment was characterized by a positive paternal transference. She began to compliment me, appreciate the value and importance of her sessions, and recognize how she looked forward to them. The sarcastic and argumentative edge had disappeared from her voice. Nonetheless, the therapy remained at a superficial level.

At this point, the patient began to experience a recrudescence of physical symptoms, which were likely delayed side effects from chemotherapy or low immune response. She developed pains in her muscles and joints, became nauseated, and had a poor appetite. She had some wheezing and shortness of breath. The patient described weakness in the morning and dizziness throughout the day. Concomitant with these symptoms, her mode of attire slowly altered—although never sloppy or ill-kempt, she dressed more informally, preferring blue jeans and casual clothes. She was less charming but much more genuine. A new phase of the therapy was thereby ushered in.

She described how upset she became when reading about people with cancer, especially young people. She was bothered by every little symptom, whereas previously no symptom had bothered her. She recalled, once again, the experience of surgery, but this time with other affects—the anesthesia, the numbing pain medication, the drowsy unreal state that was almost like a dream. She spent many sessions crying softly for the entire hour. This was not the angry pouting of a 15-year-old, but the lonely tears of a 6- or 7-year-old in the hospital. At times, she would curl up on the couch. On other occasions, she sat on the floor. She might interrupt the hour briefly to go to the bathroom and then return to the office. I found the sessions sad and poignant and at one point wondered aloud whether therapy was just adding to her pain. She insisted that it was not; on the contrary, the sessions were a great relief. She said that her behavior "on the outside" was going on almost in a normal way: she was caring for her household and her son and was going about her business as usual because she could let herself go in my office. I would give her 5 minutes' warning before the end of the session; she would then pull herself together and go to the bathroom to splash water on her face before departing. It was most reassuring to me that she was in the hands of a good oncologist who had her medical condition in full control.

Ms. E. missed one group of sessions when she became bedridden with bad sweats and nausea. Other than that, despite her many symptoms, she attended regularly. During the "bad times," she might sit in my waiting room after the sessions reconstituting herself for 10 or 15 minutes by reading magazines. I permitted this parameter, and it was not abused. I specifically avoided the role of oncologist, letting her own physician totally assume this function. This made it possible to hear her reactions to medical care, both favorable and unfavorable, without becoming a party to them.

Her physical condition continued to deteriorate, with one low-grade infection after another. As she became more vulnerable physically, she underwent a parallel regression psychologically in the therapy. The patient was undergoing a regression in the classic sense of the word, becoming more infantile, not more primitive. She described terrible nausea and vomiting, fevers, and how every bone and joint in her body ached. She remained exhausted and required iron supplementation and other medications. She had a dream: *I'm in a garage, lying down. My husband is waxing a new Alfa Romeo. I have only a broken-down Volvo.* She felt that she was the Volvo; her husband was with another woman, perhaps someone who he found more desirable. The garage was the hospital where chemotherapy takes place. She was tearful. She said she felt tired out. She wondered whether "Volvo" and "vagina" had some connection. She said that her mother had felt that the use of the mind was not for women. Her images were of the bad mother who let her suffer. She spoke of a friend who died at age 23 from cancer. She wondered whether this would not have been the easier way out. These sessions were at the lowest ebb of her despair.

During this period of indolent physical symptoms and psychological regression, Ms. E. was thrust into the midst of a maternal transference with the cherishing mother she had always hoped for. The illness permitted not only a return to that state but an "excuse" to vocalize the pain and loneliness in a way not permitted as a child, or too well defended against as an adult. My acceptance of this behavior encouraged her to go deeper. She had a striking dream fragment of a mother chimpanzee grooming its baby. Grooming was a sign of love, and being dressed up was the only maternal sign she recalled from her mother. But it was an intimate, almost medical, kind of attention— removal of lice equated with removal of cancer as an act of love without being repelled. A month later, she had another dream: *I was at a grave. A man downstairs was at a child's birthday. I went upstairs and began cooking for my friend Mr. F.* She said that she felt she saw that the way to overcome her despair was to grow up (go upstairs) and to leave the child's birthday party. She must begin to think of people other than herself (symbolized by cooking for a friend).

When the transference to her mother was most intense, she had the realization that she was a mother herself! She began to think of her son's needs as an individual and separate personality.

As soon as she felt better, Ms. E. enrolled her son at a nursery school. At the same time, she decided to return to school herself. This would be a second chance, really the first chance, to use her mind. She said she did not want to reassume the role of a charming plaything. She realized that women, not only men, have minds. So the idea for her son's education and her own reeducation began concurrently. Proudly, she reported an A on her first exam some months later.

In time, Ms. E.'s physical symptoms gradually abated, and she emerged from the regressive state. She was pleased that she could be more sober and mature. She said she had to rely on herself ultimately and not on any other person and made plans to continue her education. She began to speak of termination, and her motivation for intensive work diminished. Noting her decreasing motivation, I agreed and a date was set.

As termination approached, she had a dream: *My house is a hospital. Albert Einstein is sitting in a chair. I am sitting by his feet on the ottoman.* Her associations led to the therapist. She said that I had helped her as Einstein might have, by great intelligence. She said I understood her, that she used to present herself as less distressed than she really was. My realization of this had allowed her to start a new life. For the first time, she was in a setting where she could be honest about how she felt, about anything. She ended the therapy with a sense of gratitude and genuine warmth.

As treatment ended, the transference had returned to a paternal one— I was the intelligent, devoted, early father who would support her academic study. This transference was left untouched. It was on that sanguine note that the therapy ended.

Comment

Ms. E. suffered early abandonment by both her parents. Her father "left her" after his stroke when she was 7, and her mother, affectively, from her earliest childhood. These abandonments led to personality characteristics of pseudoindependence. She developed the view that life was a game and didn't really count. She was able to maintain this adaptation and to have her various needs satisfied because of her wit, charm, and beauty. Her marriage to an older, well-to-do, established man was a compromise. It met her manifest needs for attention and material goals, but, even so, she had a nagging sense that she could be more and take less. Her mind, really her sense of self, had been neglected. The denial was adaptive, and, because she was action prone rather than reflective, it is doubtful that she would ever have found her way into a therapist's consulting room. Conceivably, this could have occurred in late middle age when her attractiveness was less dazzling and when she couldn't run so fast. Kernberg (1987) suggested that some patients may be less prone to acting out in their treatment if the treatment is initiated in middle age. The older patient's awareness of long-standing cycles of idealization and devaluation may foster emotional introspection and motivation to change. There is a need to accept imperfection in others and in the self. Some patients who consult with therapists in their late 40s or early 50s may have a better prognosis than those seen in their 20s and 30s.

The denial was adaptive as well during the acute phase of Ms. E.'s illness and surgery. But as she was recovering, an acute illness became a chronic one. The illness slowed her down and demanded that she think about her life rather than merely react to it.

Although similar patients without medical illness do arrive in the psychiatrist's office, they are more difficult to reach. They often devalue and disparage, or are sensitive to criticism, and refuse to be touched by the therapeutic experience. A trusting regression is often not possible. They usually leave after a few sessions and search for magical solutions elsewhere. However, with this patient, the sapping debility of her illness and its physical effects facilitated a slowdown and permitted the necessary regression and introspection. The grief and the sadness of her early affective deprivation could then emerge for the first time.

Only then, having been through the crucible and having come through it annealed, could she begin to take on new adaptations and new identifications. She was able to appreciate her father's sober devotion to his work. Even her mother could be reconciled with and at least partially forgiven; selfish, talented, and yet fiercely independent, her mother had qualities that she might admire.

The fact that Ms. E. had sufficient ego strength to reconstitute herself after each session allowed the therapy to proceed. The fact that her disease was improving rather than on a downhill course allowed her life to proceed.

It was necessary to maintain a psychodynamic posture throughout to allow these various dramas to unfold. I believe that these results would have been unattainable if a purely supportive psychotherapy had been attempted. This, in a way, was just what the patient had extracted from men throughout her life, and the therapy would have been merely a repetitive experience rather than an opportunity for growth.

At the time of termination, Ms. E. had achieved certain intrapsychic goals; life goals would have to await clarification of her medical status. Psychotherapy was able to take a major physical illness and turn it from just a catastrophe into an opportunity as well.

Other opportunities and life events at some future time would have to provide the motivation for any further work.

Discussion

When medical or surgical catastrophes occur, many patients who are otherwise resistant to psychodynamic psychotherapy can be reached by it. These reality crises force individuals to reevaluate their lives and take stock. Serious illness also facilitates the kind of regression that permits self-reflection and self-examination in the therapeutic setting. Yet, working so closely and so intensively with chronically ill patients is bound to arouse countertransference feelings in the therapist.

Countertransference

I made the assumption right from the start, with no good evidence to support it, that Ms. E. was not a dying patient. Having previously treated two terminally ill patients, I recalled the personal toll that these treatments exacted from me. Ms. E. was taken on as someone who had been seriously ill but who had been cured. Happily, I was correct, but this attitude on my part was wishful thinking.

My avoidance of contact with her oncologist was possibly psychotherapeutically sound but more likely was a defensive maneuver on my part. I had no evidence that the emergence of her physical symptoms was merely a side effect of her chemotherapy rather than a recurrence of the illness, and reassuring myself that "she was in the hands of a good oncologist who had her medical condition in full control" was pure surmise.

Even the dream where she was at a grave and then went upstairs to see Mr. F. might have been seen in other ways. I did not think of the alternative interpretation that she might be going "upstairs" to Heaven to join her father.

In a classic article on countertransference problems of psychiatrists who treat medically ill patients, Mendelson and Meyer (1961) described the expression of fixed and relatively unconscious anxiety-determined responses to the patient as the hallmark of countertransference. These responses may interfere with the therapist's clinical judgment. Every therapist, like every other human being, has his or her own concerns about chronic illness, helplessness, and death. The therapist especially cannot hide behind the technical and procedure-oriented tasks of most physicians and is exposed to the full volume of the patient's despair, anxiety, and anger.

Mushatt (1978) stated that the countertransference problems aroused by these physically ill patients afford the most powerful motivation to see them as untreatable by psychodynamic psychotherapy. He further suggested that a common denial often exists between therapist and patient regarding the severity of the condition of the patient once a psychodynamic psychotherapy has begun: each minimizes the severity to protect the other. I discussed patients' denial in Chapter 3; the therapist's denial is countertransference.

A moving account of the treatment of dying patients was described by Norton (1963). She felt that an essential prerequisite of psychodynamic psychotherapy is consciously accepting "countertransference." That is, seriously ill patients confront the therapist with guilt and injuries to his or her own narcissism—the therapist cannot cure everyone. These patients become a constant reminder of the therapist's own limitations. Undue defenses on therapists' part against these painful affects may unfortunately distance them from patients, just when patients need them most. The therapist has to embrace the patient's pain.

To Stop or to Go Forward

Deutsch (1945) implied that pregnant women made poor analysands: the attachments invested in the fetus and the self would leave little for an analysis. The birth of children, death of a spouse, and serious intercurrent illness have been regarded as impediments to psychodynamic psychotherapy for the same reason.

I strongly disagree. Norton's patient began to repeat and rework early aspects of her relationship with her mother in much the same way that my patient did. Ms. E. also became intensely interested in the schooling of her young child, as did Norton's patient during a brief remission. Norton concluded that one way to cope with a serious illness is to learn to give what one had not received and to overcome self-preoccupation by altruistic caring for others.

It is important to recall that Ms. E.'s body image was basically sound; her body was an instrument to be kept in good working order much like an automobile. Her body was something she knew she could rely on. When she first entered treatment, she spoke in terms of clothes, cars, and grooming (as in her dreams). When illness struck, she felt that her body was out of whack rather than fundamentally defective; she just had to find the right way to repair it. As treatment progressed, there was a sadness at the loss of function but no self-pity or angry "Why me's." I had great admiration for her pluck and courage throughout.

In a questionnaire study that colleagues and I conducted many years back (Druss et al. 1969) of patients who underwent a colectomy for bowel cancer, I was struck then, as I am today, that these individuals fell into two groups. One group was so depressed, so angry at their fate, so filled with self-pity that they ruined whatever life they had left. And most were cured! The other group grieved, then slowly learned the mechanics of the colostomy and moved on to continue their lives with optimism.

I have treated many other patients with serious medical illness, some of whom were terminally ill. One stands in admiration of their bravery in the face of adversity that appears to be all but overwhelming. What characterizes these people who can snatch some measure of victory from the very jaws of defeat? A crucial element appears to be the *absence* of the deep sense of betrayal that I discussed earlier. On the other hand, narcissistic patients ultimately turn their anger against themselves, with corresponding bitterness, depression, and lowered self-esteem.

The illness must be seen as an interruption of a life trajectory and as an event occurring in an individual with a unique history. Viederman and Perry (1980) and Viederman (1983), in their two compelling articles on the psychodynamic life narrative, described this phenomenon well. Although their case studies are a model for brief and acute intervention in a liaison psychiatry setting, their approach and overall thesis can be extended to patients in a psychodynamic psychotherapy. The therapy addresses itself to ancient betrayals symbolically replicated in the reality of the current illness. It heals old wounds and permits reconciliation to a new life trajectory.

The moment of vulnerability is also the moment of greatest susceptibility to change. Ms. E. was able to make a midcourse correction in her life trajectory. Moves in the direction of lowered expectation and altruism were facilitated as the past was almost literally relived. A body focus was expanded to include a mind focus as well; this focus hastened the sublimation of anger and undid some of the sense of childhood abandonments that had unconsciously guided her for much of her life.

She was able to rework her grief regarding the serious, potentially life-threatening illness and loss of health. This loss was a replay of early losses, and therapy had to concentrate on the betrayal of the golden fantasy in which "all losses are restored, all sorrows end."

References

Deutsch H: Pregnancy, in The Psychology of Women, Vol 2. New York, Grune & Stratton, 1945, pp 126–201

Druss RG: Cryptorchism and body image: the psychoanalysis of a case. J Am Psychoanal Assoc 26:69–85, 1978

Druss RG, O'Connor J, Stern L: Psychologic response to colectomy, II: adjustment to a permanent colostomy. Arch Gen Psychiatry 20:419–427, 1969

Fawzy F, Causius N, Fawzy N, et al: A structured psychiatric intervention for cancer patients, I: changes over time in methods of coping and affective disturbance. Arch Gen Psychiatry 47:720–725, 1990

Fawzy F, Fawzy N, Hyun C, et al: Malignant melanoma: effects of an early structured psychiatric intervention, coping, and affective state on recurrence and survival 6 years later. Arch Gen Psychiatry 50:681–689, 1993

Finkel J: Psychotherapy in medical practice, in Psychiatric Management for Medical Practitioners. Edited by Kornfeld D, Finkel J. New York, Grune & Stratton, 1982, pp 47–60

Gabbard GO: Psychodynamic psychiatry in the "decade of the brain." Am J Psychiatry 149:991–998, 1992

Gabbard GO: Psychodynamic Psychiatry in Clinical Practice, 2nd Edition. Washington, DC, American Psychiatric Press, 1994

Garber L: Transformations in self-understandings in surgeons whose treatment efforts were not successful. Am J Psychother 44:75–84, 1990

Greer S, Mooney S, Baruch J: Evaluation of adjuvant psychological therapy for clinically referred cancer patients. Br J Cancer 63:257–260, 1991

Haag A: Psychosomatic consultation-liaison service in a medical outpatient department: experience with a random sample of patients. Psychother Psychosom 42:205–212, 1984

Karush A, Daniels GE: Ulcerative colitis: the psychoanalysis of two cases. Psychosom Med 15:140–167, 1953

Kernberg O: Pathologic narcissism in middle age, in Internal Worlds and External Realities. Northvale, NJ, Jason Aronson, 1987, pp 135–153

Levitan S, Kornfeld D: Clinical and cost benefits of liaison psychiatry. Am J Psychiatry 138:790–795, 1981

Margolin S: The behavior of the stomach during psychoanalysis. Psychoanal Q 20:349–373, 1951

Mendelson M, Meyer E: Countertransference problems of the liaison psychiatrist. Psychosom Med 23:115–122, 1961

Mushatt C: Countertransference in the treatment of patients with organic illness or major physical handicaps. Paper presented at the Discussion Group on Psychoanalytic Considerations About Patients With Organic Injury, American Psychoanalytic Association, New York, December 1978

Norton J: Treatment of a dying patient. Psychoanal Study Child 18:541–560, 1963

Schindler B, Shook J, Schwartz G: Beneficial effects of psychiatric intervention after coronary artery bypass graft surgery. Gen Hosp Psychiatry 11:358–364, 1989

Sperling M: Transference neurosis in patients with psychoanalytic disorders. Psychoanal Q 36:342–355, 1967

Strain J, Grossman S: Psychologic Care of the Mentally Ill: A Primer in Liaison Psychiatry. New York, Appleton-Century-Crofts, 1975

Viederman M: The psychodynamic life narrative: a psychotherapeutic intervention useful in crisis situations. Psychiatry 46:236–246, 1983

Viederman M, Perry S: Use of a psychodynamic life narrative in the treatment of depression in the physically ill. Gen Hosp Psychiatry 3:177–185, 1980

5

Treatment Philosophy

A t the end of each chapter of this section, I have made passing and somewhat hurried references to treatment. I would like to take the opportunity now, in a somewhat more organized and leisurely way, to summarize various recommendations and to describe a treatment philosophy. The four main positions I emphasize are 1) empathy and the subjective experience of the patient, 2) the need for flexibility, 3) the historical perspective, and 4) therapeutic optimism.

Empathy and the Subjective Experience of the Patient

When I am treating a patient with a medical condition, I read everything I can about that disease, the various options for treatment, and its course and prognosis. I listen carefully to the concerns and opinions of the referring physicians. However, medically sick patients still need one place they can go and speak their minds about the disease, its care, and what it all means to them. I have seen patients who have idealized their internist or surgeon, or despised him or her, or even a few who erotized the encounter. Psychiatrists must regard all of these reports as emerging from the subjective world of the patient that they alone are privileged to enter. In return, the therapist gives the patient empathy and understanding. In fact, the *American Heritage Dictionary* defines empathy as "an understanding so intimate that the feelings, thoughts, and motives of one are readily comprehended by another" (p. 603).

This treatment approach is clearly enunciated by the Group for the Advancement of Psychiatry (1993): "the second meaning of empathy [is] an attitude of benevolent helpfulness; a selectively tuned concern for the other; a willingness to 'stand alongside' the patient, valuing the patient as a person and accepting the legitimacy of the patient's feeling and ideas whatever they may be" (p. 22). This excellent report, *Caring for People With Physical Impairment: The Journey Back*, depicts the whole process of rehabilitation as an odyssey in which a variety of caregivers accompany each patient along part of this metaphorical journey. The group remarks that "the reader will soon notice the heavy emphasis given to subjective experience in this work" (p. 6) and stresses that the caregiver needs to be ready to experience the subjective world of the patient as the two work together.

One exception to this subjective stance would, of course, be the emergence of life-and-death situations. If a female patient tells me she has discovered a breast lump but hopes it is of no account and will go away, I would initially discuss her fears (surgery? disfigurement? pain? death?) and hope that the insights gained would lead her to seek an evaluation. But I wouldn't give her too much time. If her denial was so great, or her reality testing so poor, as to lead to continued inaction, I would demand that she call, from my office if necessary, to make an appointment with a surgeon; and I would follow through every step of the way, as I would with any potentially self-destructive act. Some years ago, I was treating a person with brittle diabetes who became hypoglycemic during a session. I grabbed her and rushed her to the local diner. After I got a large glass of orange juice into her, I called her husband to take her home and to call her internist. We spent the next few months discussing what led this usually meticulous woman to double her usual dose of insulin that morning, and the treatment progress was accelerated by her self-created crisis. These are proper responses to temporary crises, but the empathic search for subjective truth still remains the ongoing goal.

Flexibility

Whenever I undertake psychotherapy with medically ill patients, I am prepared to be flexible in my approach to their care. Every patient is different, and, as seen in other chapters, each will follow his or her own path to physical health. More important, however, is the enormous variability in state of health over time for any given patient.

It is the nature of medical illness that there are periods of quiescence during which in-depth psychodynamic work can be done and periods of rapid change during which other measures are required. The patient may go through many cycles of medical exacerbation and remission, and the psychiatrist must vary the technique accordingly and not squeeze the patient into a preset therapeutic mold. Any therapist wedded to a single modality, either ideologically or by training, should not undertake these cases.

For some patients, a full analysis (Druss 1978) or psychodynamic psychotherapy is not only possible but is the treatment of choice. I presented the case of such a patient in Chapter 4. But even here, the therapist must be prepared to shift gears if there is a crisis (like the above-mentioned hypoglycemia). With appropriate modifications, the therapy need not be derailed by an exacerbation, or surgery, or new medical treatment but can go on. Telephone sessions conducted properly, even from a hospital bed, are often a fine substitute for unavoidable absences. With or without these telephone sessions, the continuity of therapy can often be preserved even through a medical crisis. (Therapists do this all the time in the treatment of women undergoing childbirth.) I have visited medically ill patients at the hospital bedside and conducted brief sessions in their homes during acute crises. These sessions were helpful and illuminating and did not interfere with a full psychodynamic therapy when the patient was better.

I subscribe to the concept of boundaries in clinical practice regarding location of treatment, clearly elucidated by Gutheil and Gabbard (1993). These home or hospital visits have been few and have been reserved for severe medical exacerbations. The presence of a coexisting medical illness alone is no reason to violate any therapeutic boundaries, and flexibility is never to be construed as license.

Even if the patient has been well selected, psychodynamic psychotherapy may not be the best treatment modality because of an error in timing. I have had sophisticated, high-functioning patients who have fled the offices of orthodox analysts who would not or could not temporarily abandon the classical model. One patient described an analysis that continued unchanged even though he was experiencing and describing chest pains on the couch. Good psychodynamic work was done after he had his coronary bypass, but he remained horrified that he had been required to free-associate about increasing chest pain during the daily sessions with his former analyst.

During periods of exacerbation, cognitive therapies (Barsky 1992; Beck et al. 1979; Greer et al. 1991) and support (Massie and Holland 1990) are often more helpful. These require greater activity and more presence on the part of the therapist. During such phases, a free-association treatment may actually be counterproductive and only serve to increase self-preoccupation and despondency. When the patient needs to act, to face surgery, or to try a new medication, etc., the therapist is often best advised to use the cognitive-behavioral method of treatment.

Depression accompanies many medical illnesses. Cassem (1991) reported that psychiatric consultants to a medical ward will make a diagnosis of major depression in about 20% of the patients they see and that there is often a resurgence of depression shortly after a patient is discharged to home and faces the long, slow task of recuperation. According to Hall et al. (1987), certain physical conditions (including Parkinson's disease, hypothyroidism, multiple sclerosis, pancreatic cancer, and various viral infections) appear to add a physiological component to the depression as well as the reactive psychological component. Ever since the reports of sudden death associated with amitriptyline hydrochloride in cardiac patients, psychiatrists have been reluctant to make use of familiar tricyclic antidepressants to treat patients with intercurrent medical diseases. But, as Federoff and Robinson (1989) stressed, "although the use of antidepressant medication requires caution, the treatment of depression in patients with stroke may result in significant physical and cognitive recovery, as well as improvement in their emotional state" (p. 18).

In part to clarify this complex state of affairs, Roose and Glassman (1989) reviewed the effects of tricyclics on pulse, blood pressure, rhythm, and cardiac conduction in patients with and without heart disease, and they also discussed the newer nontricyclic antidepressants. Their detailed findings and practical suggestions for treatment are beyond the scope of this volume, and I refer the reader to this excellent monograph for guidance. The advent of the selective serotonin reuptake inhibitors (SSRIs) has augmented the repertoire of psychiatrists who treat depressed medically ill patients. The current *Drug Evaluations Annual* of the American Medical Association (1994) states that the SSRIs "do not possess significant sedative, anticholinergic, or hypotensive effects; do not have significant effects on cardiac conduction" (p. 298). Drugs like fluoxetine, sertraline, and paroxetine may be "particularly useful in patients with concurrent illness such as hypertension, coronary artery disease, prostatic enlargement . . . and in the elderly" (p. 298). I send my own patients who have depression that is complicated by cardiovascular disease or who are taking other prescription drugs and need antidepressant medication to a trusted psychopharmacologist for consultation and initiation of drug therapy. But each reader should judge his or her training and competence in this area and act accordingly; do not let your own ignorance be the limiting factor.

The psychiatrist should be open to the concomitant use of adjunctive treatments done by others. I describe later, in Chapter 8, "Exercise, Well-Being, and Restoration," dramatic improvements in postcoronary patients when they attended organized exercise programs; mental as well as physical health improved. I never scoff at anyone who wishes to see a physical therapist, an acupuncturist, a hypnotist for pain, etc., as long as the data from these encounters are grist for one's own mill. These therapists and their treatments are not to be dismissed as competitors for us nor should the patient's choosing to consult with them be considered resistance on the patient's part.

I cannot emphasize enough the value of mutual aid groups such as Alcoholics Anonymous, Smoke Enders, Weight Watchers, Reach for Recovery (cancer), and the Ileostomy Society. Twenty-five years after treating that young woman with an ileostomy described in the "Introduction," I am all the more convinced that an enthusiastic referral to such a group may be the best service we can perform for many of these patients.

Certain corrective surgical procedures seem to be more than mere whitewash and superficial camouflage; they can lead to fundamental changes in ego structure and body image. The regressive aspects of surgery mimic the childhood state when the ego was first being formed, and the body image in adulthood is more fluid than previously realized. Elsewhere I described the dramatically positive psychological effects of augmentation breast surgery (Druss 1973) and the correction of undescended testes by orchidopexy (Druss 1978). The young woman described in Chapter 2 with a cleft palate turned from a ridiculed child to a sociable teenager when her fear of corrective surgery was overcome and she could benefit from the corrective procedure. When individuals with somatic delusions are carefully excluded and there is a clear need, many patients with psychological problems can benefit from cosmetic surgery. Therapists should be flexible here as well, and these opportunities should be gently and tactfully explored.

In the spirit of flexibility, I wish to say a few words about family and couples therapy for medically ill patients. Few traumas are so devastating to the ecology of a family as the severe sickness of one of its members. I don't think it is possible to treat a medically ill person without taking note of the tormented relative(s) suffering behind the scenes. Imagine, if you will, a man whose beloved wife is deteriorating over a decade's time with multiple sclerosis. Imagine the love, pity, and grief, as well as the anger and sense of being trapped, and the ensuing guilt, that are his daily bread. Think as well of a worried wife whose husband, the sole breadwinner, has been struck by a coronary and is demoralized and unable to provide for either her or himself.

The effect of men's heart disease on their wives has been well discussed by Shanfield (1990). He found high levels of psychological distress in the spouses and described a psychosocial crisis in the entire family. He recommended direct intervention with those wives at risk and including them in the rehabilitation process as much as possible.

Lear (1980), in her book *Heartsounds,* brought all the skills of a superb reporter to bear on her account of her own husband's downhill course. The book begins with his sudden myocardial infarction when she was in Europe, goes on to describe his open-heart surgery to correct a ventricular aneurysm and his enduring every possible postoperative complication, explains his partial recovery impaired by memory defects, and then accounts his eventual death. The reader wonders along the way, who is suffering more—the designated patient or the loving author? Both.

In December of 1956, Niall O'Casey, the much loved son of Sean and Eileen O'Casey, died at age 21 of leukemia. The following April, Sean, a playwright, began a secret diary and made weekly entries in it, sometimes a single word and sometimes a short essay. It is clear from reading *Niall: A Lament* (1991) that his overwhelming grief did not lessen with the passage of time and life's outer successes. His wife published this heartrending diary years after O'Casey himself had died, and every page shows the poet's hand, and the poet's heart.

Psychiatrists who treat medically ill patients must make use of all therapeutic techniques available. Nadelson and Polonsky (1989) described the uses and techniques of couples therapy and made the point that "technique must also be separated from theory, so that restrictions that come out of

dogma rather than clinical indicators do not cloud the therapist's understanding" (p. 1550). Although not directly referring to a medical illness,
they go on to say that "a spouse is affected not only by the partner's disorder,
but also by the partner's treatment" (p. 1551), and their instructions regarding the mentally ill apply equally to the medically ill.

Gabbard (1994) devoted a section of his text to family and marital therapy, describing the various theoretical orientations, indications, and techniques. He warned of the strong countertransferences evoked in family
therapies, and I only add that treatments in which one member is seriously
ill are no exception. It is rare in my work with medically ill patients that I do
not make use of family therapy somewhere along the way as the indications
present themselves, most often in the evaluation phase or at a time of crisis.

I hypothesized in Chapter 2, "Hypochondriasis in Medically Ill Patients," that the ongoing presence of a sick person in the household can be
traumatic to a very young and noncomprehending child, who may need to
be shielded prophylactically. In contrast, an older child or adolescent may
want to participate in both the care and comfort of an afflicted parent.

In other situations, a spouse, parent, or child of the patient may need
his or her own therapist. In this case, I feel that a separate referral to a col-
league is indicated. The relative may have to learn to separate from the patient and develop his or her own life. Both parties will benefit when each
has his or her own safe haven.

Historical Perspective

I begin any therapy of a medically ill patient with a good personal history.
The history need not be long or taken chronologically, but certain elements should be covered.

A description of the disease in the patient's own words is a useful starting place because it is what is on his or her mind. It immediately builds
rapport. It also allows the therapist to begin to understand the patient's
various attitudes toward the illness.

A history of the individual's childhood, with special emphasis on childhood illnesses and physical traumas, should be included. As I described in
Chapter 2, the health of those who are near and dear to the patient must
also be ascertained. Some of these data may be repressed or unavailable

initially and emerge only as the therapy progresses, but an initial effort can often be rewarding.

Comments about patients' own views about their physical selves should accompany the historical narrative. Did the patient perceive himself or herself as damaged, deformed, or defective even before the current illness began? Is the disease viewed as a punishment and a depressive cast given to the description? Does the patient state quite openly, "Why me?" and "What have I done to deserve this?" Inquiries regarding narcissistic entitlement and the patient's expectation for a perfect, unafflicted life can then be made. The sense that the disease is a betrayal of an unwritten and unspoken contract with parents will then emerge, and therapists know they are in for a long and difficult time.

Was the patient sickly and able to gain attention for the "sick role" during childhood? A cognitive-behavioral approach might be undertaken to help the patient "unlearn" this mode of adaptation and to "learn" a more positive and assertive outlook. The rewards of fitness and mastery can be introduced.

Throughout this book, I stress the importance of brave or stoical parents who reward these characteristics in their children as forerunners of future resiliency. I would try to determine if these characteristics exist in either of the patient's parents by a brief character sketch of each parent elicited from the patient and to determine how much of this attitude was introjected by the patient. If the patient has introjected such attitudes, insight-oriented therapies and transference analysis may be more likely to be of use for at least certain phases of the treatment.

I make an additional evaluation at the start of the treatment: my own judgment about the competence and adequacy of the medical care being given. Only if I am fully comfortable that the primary care is sound can I take the position of psychodynamic subjectivity that I initially suggested. If not, the patient must be helped to assert dissatisfaction and to get proper medical care. The patient's real life-support system is equally crucial, whether it be spouse, parents, children, or friends.

We should also be interested in the immediate history proximate to the outbreak or emergence of a disease. Some diseases may be directly precipitated by stress in the workplace or the home, and the therapy might consist of nothing more than helping the patient extract himself or herself from a stressful environment.

Much more often, the illness itself is the trigger, and our task is a more lengthy and complex psychodynamic one—the search with the patient for the neurotic infrastructure, which ultimately emanates from childhood experiences, that gives undue power and dread to the presenting disease. The "history" then will unfold throughout the entire therapeutic encounter.

Optimism

Maintaining an optimistic attitude is absolutely crucial in working with these patients. This attitude includes a belief in the body's natural power to heal itself when unencumbered by either medical insult or neurosis and that the physician's role—any physician, psychiatrist included—is ultimately to facilitate self-healing. It also includes a belief that the worst scenario rarely occurs. Medically ill patients are always playing with statistics and odds. Most biopsies are negative, most lumps are not cancer, and most examinations are normal. Disasters, when they occur, come from unexpected and unlikely sources, rarely the ones anticipated and feared and overprepared for.

No matter how sick or desperate, everyone is capable of some choice in how he or she feels. This statement may seem illogical or at the very least paradoxical, but humans are endowed with some element of choice in the perceptions of their outer and inner worlds—including how they feel. One is mindful of the Hebrew Bible, which preached long ago, "I have given you this day blessing and curse, life and death: choose life" (Deuteronomy 30:19).

Arnold Cooper (1986), in an article discussing therapeutic effectiveness in psychoanalysis, advised, "The analyst cannot do his job well if he is not basically optimistic and dedicated to the work he is conducting. The patient must perceive that the analyst is not easily discouraged, is extraordinarily persistent, and will stick by the patient no matter what" (p. 577).

So much more the case in working with physical illness. It is no fun to be sick. In addition to their understanding and therapeutic work, psychiatrists treating medically ill patients must manifest their optimism, not about the patient's course or ultimate prognosis, which no one knows, but about the patient's courage, no matter what the outcome.

References

American Heritage Dictionary of the English Language, 3rd Edition. Boston, MA, Houghton Mifflin, 1992

Barsky A: Amplification, somatization and the somatoform disorders. Psychosomatics 33:28–34, 1992

Beck A, Rush AJ, Shaw B, et al: Cognitive Therapy of Depression. New York, Guilford, 1979

Cassem N (ed): Depression, in Massachusetts General Hospital Handbook of General Hospital Psychiatry, 3rd Edition. St. Louis, MO, Mosby Year Book, 1991, pp 237–268

Cooper A: Some limitations on therapeutic effectiveness: the "burnout syndrome" in psychoanalysts. Psychoanal Q 55:576–598, 1986

Drug Evaluations Annual. Chicago, IL, American Medical Association, 1994

Druss RG: Changes in body image following augmentation breast surgery. International Journal of Psychoanalysis and Psychotherapy 2:248–256, 1973

Druss RG: Cryptorchism and body image: the psychoanalysis of a case. J Am Psychoanal Assoc 26:69–85, 1978

Federoff J, Robinson R: Tricyclic antidepressants in the treatment of post-stroke depression. J Clin Psychiatry 50 (suppl):18–23, 1989

Gabbard G: Psychodynamic Psychiatry in Clinical PracticeL The DSM-IV Edition. Washington, DC, American Psychiatric Press, 1994

Greer S, Moorey S, Baruch J: Evaluation of adjuvant psychological therapy for clinically referred cancer patients. Br J Cancer 63:257–260, 1991

Group for the Advancement of Psychiatry: Caring for People With Physical Impairment: The Journey Back (Report 135). Washington, DC, American Psychiatric Press, 1993

Gutheil T, Gabbard G: The concept of boundaries in clinical practice: theoretical and risk-management dimensions. Am J Psychiatry 150:188–196, 1993

Hall R, Beresford T, Blow F: Depression and medical illness: an overview, in Presentations of Depression: Depression in Medical and Other Psychiatric Disorders. Edited by Cameron O. New York, Wiley, 1987, pp 401–414

Lear M: Heartsounds. New York, Simon & Schuster, 1980

Massie MJ, Holland JCB: Depression and the cancer patient. J Clin Psychiatry 51 (suppl):7–12, 1990

Nadelson C, Polonsky DC: Couples therapy, in Comprehensive Textbook of Psychiatry/V, 5th Edition. Edited by Kaplan HI, Sadock BJ. Baltimore, MD, Williams & Wilkins, 1989, pp 1550–1556

O'Casey S: Niall: A Lament. New York, Riverrun Press, 1991

Roose S, Glassman A: Cardiovascular effects of tricyclic antidepressants in depressed patients. Journal of Clinical Psychiatry Monograph 7:1–18, 1989

Shanfield S: Myocardial infarction and patient's wives. Psychosomatics 31:138–145, 1990

II

Health

6

~~~~~~~~~~~~~~~~~~~~~~~~~

Healthy Denial

In Chapter 3, I explored pathological denial of illness in two patients who allowed their physical disease to progress to advanced stages then had unexpected negative reactions to successful medical treatment. In this chapter, I discuss people who did surprisingly well psychologically in the face of serious illness and disability. In the first vignette, I describe a patient treated by me during the last years of a terminal illness who approached her death with bravery and resoluteness. The second is based on autobiographical writings of a man with an acute, life-threatening illness (a heart attack) whose optimistic attitude strongly influenced his illness and its treatment (Cousins 1979, 1983). The third vignette is about a woman with congenital absence of the arms whose care of herself and her husband and children was dramatically depicted on the television program *60 Minutes* (1981). Extrapolating from these very different situations, I consider what these individuals had in common that enabled them to function effectively and maintain a high degree of optimism confronting adversity and where they might have acquired these adaptive traits. I also reexamine the concept of positive denial and speculate on its role in their healthy response to illness and disability.

Portions of this chapter are adapted by permission of the publisher from Druss RG, Douglas CJ: "Adaptive Responses to Illness and Disability: Healthy Denial." *General Hospital Psychiatry* 10:163–168, 1988. Copyright 1988 by Elsevier Science Publishing Co., Inc.

Case Reports

Case 1

Ms. N. was a 51-year-old, single, decorating editor of a major fashion magazine. She had metastatic breast cancer and was receiving biweekly chemotherapy, which had already resulted in hair loss and premature menopause. She said she entered psychotherapy because she wanted to be in better shape psychologically for the man with whom she was living. She was attractive and dressed with such flair and style that one hardly noticed the obligatory kerchief covering her total alopecia.

She knew full well that she had at most 1 or 2 good years left and was determined to make the most of them. Her spirits were usually good despite the continuing and realistic horror of the chemotherapy injections. She did not become overtly depressed when she later had to undergo an adrenalectomy and oophorectomy or when severe osteoporosis eventually left her in constant pain. Although she was never able to have a much hoped for reconstructive mammoplasty, she did have a face-lift to "cheer up her lover."

Ms. N. was the younger of two children in a family from the Midwest. She adored her father, who had always been proud of her artistic achievements. He loved a good time and had imbued her with optimism and energy. She was also close to her older brother but related poorly to her mother, whom she described as shy and withdrawn. As a child, she enjoyed playing rough-and-tumble sports with boys, and she remained a tomboy until college.

Her only previous experience of serious illness was a bout of appendicitis at age 21, which developed into peritonitis and necessitated a 2-month hospitalization. Treatment with sulfa drugs resulted in total hair loss for 6 months. Ms. N. said this experience had taught her the value of self-reliance and had given her a sense of confidence in her ability to endure adversity.

Early in the course of her psychotherapy, Ms. N. bought an apple orchard in the country. As she declined physically, she made it a project to build a house in the orchard and spent weekends overseeing its construction. One day, after a weekend in the country, she came to the office in a buoyant mood. The house was finished. She had found a spot in the orchard where she could see the entire vista of her property. Seated there, because she could hardly stand, she noticed the arrival of a flock of bluebirds. She spent hours watching them build their nest, and, recounting this, she exclaimed, "I had the greatest weekend!" This attitude persisted until the very end, when she was in extremis, so severely debilitated that she could only be seen at home or in the hospital. She died quietly in the hospital 3 years after psychotherapy had begun. The only instance of self-deception about the seriousness of her condition was when she attributed her somnolence and liver function abnormalities to hepatitis rather than metastases.

Case 2

At age 65, several years after he left his position as editor of *The Saturday Review* to begin a new career as senior lecturer at the UCLA School of Medicine, Norman Cousins suffered a massive heart attack. He provided a vivid firsthand account of his experience in *The Healing Heart* (1983). Although he had been having bouts of breathlessness in the weeks preceding the attack, he had kept up a hectic schedule of travel and lecturing. At the time of the attack, short of breath, coughing up blood, and in severe pain, he joked with paramedics and refused morphine, insisting that his "own endorphins could do the job." He also convinced the ambulance driver to turn off the siren and drive at ordinary speeds to the hospital. On arrival at the emergency room, he sat up on the stretcher, grinned at his alarmed physicians, and exclaimed, "Gentlemen, I want you to know that you are looking at the darndest healing machine that's ever been wheeled into this hospital!" (Fareed 1983, p. 264).

He wrote that on awakening in the critical care unit the next morning, his first impulse was to put down notes about the events leading to the heart attack. He also began to read voraciously about heart disease and questioned the indications for every medicine prescribed. He described his predominant feelings during this time as "curiosity, a sense of challenge and confidence" (Cousins 1983, p. 53). After consultation with several cardiologists, he decided to defer coronary angiography and instead embarked on a cardiac reconditioning program of his own design. After 6 months, he agreed to undergo an exercise stress test to assess his progress but only if he could run the treadmill controls himself. The results were favorable.

A year later, despite periodic reoccurrence of symptoms, he had resumed vigorous tennis, golf, and a busy lecturing schedule.

Cousins (1983) stated that his first experience in dealing with a bleak medical diagnosis came at age 10 when he was sent to a tuberculosis sanitarium for 6 months. He recalled:

What was most interesting to me about that early experience was that patients divided themselves into two groups: those who were confident they would beat back the disease and be able to resume normal lives and those who resigned themselves to a prolonged and even fatal illness. Those of us who held to the optimistic view became good friends, involved ourselves in creative activities and had little to do with the patients who had resigned themselves to worst. . . . I couldn't help being impressed with the fact that the boys in my group had a far higher percentage of "discharged as cured" outcomes. (pp. 155–156)

After his discharge, frail and weighing only 78 pounds, Cousins invested his weekly allowance in hiring a local boy for baseball practice. Within 2 years, 6 inches taller and 40 pounds heavier, he became captain of the neighborhood baseball team. The important role played by such optimism and positive thinking in his recovery from ankylosing spondylitis at age 49 was the subject of *Anatomy of an Illness* (1979).

Cousins attributes his resilience in the face of these adversities to a strong marriage with a woman whom he sees as "endowed with a blessed cheerfulness" and to a father, a robust man, who lived until age 94.

Case 3

In May of 1981, the weekly CBS News documentary *60 Minutes* broadcast a feature called "Bonnie" about a 40-year-old woman who was born without arms. The story opened with her playing the organ with her feet and later showed her washing the dishes ("I get dishpan feet!"), dressing ("It's easier for me, I think, than a lot of women"), and driving a car ("The only time an officer asked to see my license was when I had a headlight out . . . it scared him to death!"). She told the interviewer that the only thing she could not do and really missed was bike riding with her two children.

She had corresponded with her husband for more than a year before they actually met, and she married him 3 months later. He said about their marriage, "I saw a rich philosophy in her." Although told by doctors that there was a possibility that her children might be born armless, she took the chance: "Mark was so beautiful. He was perfect, as Matthew is. And I don't think they have any hang-ups. . . . It worried me when they were little, how they would be able to adjust to me, to accept me as just Mom. So as soon as they learned to talk, we talked about me. We laughed and made jokes about me. Never was there a time when I said, 'I don't want to talk about it.'"

She lectures extensively about her experience to groups of disabled people around the country and has published an autobiography: "All of our lives we strive to be different in what we do, what we look like. And here it was just handed to me on a silver platter: I'm different." She gives her mother credit for what she has been able to accomplish: "She made me try. She made me do it. [If a handicapped child] says 'I can't,'—no, I don't know those words. They're not in my language."

Comment

These vignettes describe people who showed unusual courage confronting death, acute illness, and congenital disability. What enabled them to do well and remain optimistic in the face of such adversity? An initial comparison of the cases reveals a number of similarities that may shed light on the nature and sources of their resilience.

First, these individuals did not disavow the fact of their particular infirmity. Rather, the most threatening implications and the full emotional impact of their condition were denied. Although she knew she was going to die, Ms. N. did not see death as an immediate threat and expected to have several good years left. Depression or anxiety about her impending death was rarely experienced in a conscious way, having been displaced (attributed to the chemotherapy) or projected (her lover needed cheering up). Cousins carefully compiled the statistics on mortality following heart attacks but never believed they applied to him. He felt confident that he could beat the odds and favorably influence the course of his illness through hope and a powerful will to live. The heightened emotions that he felt during his hospitalization were experienced by him as a sense of "curiosity" or "challenge" rather than threat. Bonnie believed her armlessness had never limited her in any important way and viewed her disability almost as an enviable asset. Like Cousins, she was a risk taker; she never believed there was any chance her children would also be deformed. Without actually repudiating the fact of their disability, these individuals were able to screen out the most personally threatening consequences and focus on the positive aspects of their situations. They were people who tended to see glasses as half full rather than half empty. The resilience they showed appears to have been based at least in part on this characteristic way of seeing the world.

Another related trait they had in common was the inclination to involve themselves in creative endeavors, even in the midst of illness. As her body deteriorated, Ms. N. bought an orchard and built a house. Cousins took notes about his illnesses and turned these into best-selling books. Bonnie's efforts were directed toward raising healthy children and helping other disabled people by her example. These three individuals concentrated on generativity rather than infirmity and regarded their ailments not as a narcissistic injury but as an opportunity for personal growth. This may help explain why they were remarkably free of self-pity, anger, and envy toward those who were whole and well. They did not regard themselves as defective or damaged and seemed to retain an abiding faith in the integrity of their bodies.

Discussion

Diverse forms and degrees of denial have been described in the literature, ranging from clear-cut disavowal of illness, to keeping one's emotions about it out of awareness, to merely avoiding talking or thinking about it (Breznitz 1983; Hackett and Cassem 1974; Lazarus 1983; Perry and Viederman 1981). Whether all of these responses should properly be called "denial" has been a subject of some debate.

Once regarded as a sign of serious psychopathology, denial has been rehabilitated to the status of a "healthy" defense for patients with serious illness. The notion that positive attitudes like the "will to live" have an effect on health has been part of our conventional wisdom throughout history. Physicians from Hippocrates to Osler have attested to the *vis medicatrix naturae*, or the natural power of the body to heal itself (Dubos 1979). Modern research has now supported this popular belief.

Levy et al. (1988), using the Affect Balance Scale, which has a record of good reliability in past studies of cancer patients, found that patients with advanced cancer who reported some joy and optimism lived significantly longer than the others in their sample. In fact, the "joy factor" was the second most accurate predictor of survival time, only exceeded by "disease-free interval" in these patients.

In another study of cancer, 122 women with operable breast cancer were assessed by Dean and Surtees (1989) 3 months after operation. These authors found that those patients who used a strategy of denial had a better chance of remaining recurrence free 6–8 years later than had those women who used other coping mechanisms such as acceptance or hopelessness/helplessness. These findings with breast cancer were supported by a series of articles by Pettingale et al. (1981); a 5-year follow-up of breast cancer patients indicated the beneficial effects of denial on eventual outcome.

Levinson et al. (1989) studied 48 patients referred for treatment of unstable angina. They were divided into two groups—"high deniers" and "low deniers"—using the Hackett-Cassem Denial Scale. They found that high deniers had half as many episodes of angina during hospitalization. These authors concluded that the use of denial predicts better medical outcome during hospitalization for unstable angina. This finding confirms their 1984 study of a similar but smaller population.

Folks et al. (1988), using a modified Hackett-Cassem Denial Scale, measured preoperative denial in 121 patients scheduled for coronary bypass surgery. Their findings suggest that denial serves as an adaptive measure immediately postoperation and is predictive of improved outcome for up to 6 months after surgery.

Going beyond cancer and heart disease, Peterson et al. (1988) showed that individuals who explain bad events pessimistically at age 25 would endure poor health at ages 45–60, including more doctor visits, more infectious diseases, and lowered immune function. Locke (1982) reviewed the research on the relationship of stress, emotions, and adaptation to human immune function. He concluded that stress coupled with poor coping can lead to immunosuppressive deterioration. Scheier and Carver (1987) supported the studies by Locke. The link between optimism and faster rate of recovery from coronary bypass surgery is one of their most striking findings. There can no longer be doubts as to the benefits of healthy denial in medical illness.

The issue I wish to address is whether "healthy denial," clearly at work in the patients I described, fully explains and accounts for their singular optimism in the face of adversity. If their morale remained good, was it only because they were deceiving themselves in some way? Or are there other dimensions to, and precursors of, such optimism that the concept of "healthy denial" does not adequately encompass?

Behavior that is interpreted as "denial" may be understood in a variety of ways depending on one's conceptual orientation. Thus, what is viewed as denial from a psychodynamic perspective might be described from a cognitive viewpoint as "selective information processing" or "practicing positive mental attitudes"—threatening facts, rather than being excluded from awareness, simply receive relatively less attention, whereas positive information is placed in the foreground. From a different viewpoint, Beisser (1979) pointed out that what Hackett and colleagues regarded as evidence of denial, such as flirting with danger or risk taking, could be described within the framework of humanistic psychology as attributes of the "self-actualizing" or health-affirming person. Hence, the purely psychodynamic paradigm may ignore important dimensions of patients that enable them to feel well and function effectively when confronting disabling illness.

In a related line of investigation, social psychologists have recently become interested in whether certain personality dispositions help keep people who are under stress physically healthy. Kobasa and colleagues proposed that a particular constellation of personality characteristics that they call "hardiness" helps to buffer the illness—and reduce the effects of stressful life events (1982, 1983). The general characteristics of the "hardy" personality, as defined by these investigators, are 1) control—the belief that one can actively influence the events of one's experience, 2) commitment—an ability to feel deeply involved in or committed to one's activities, and 3) challenge—the anticipation of change as an exciting challenge to further development. It will readily be apparent that many of the personality characteristics of the patients we presented (e.g., activity versus passivity, adventuresomeness, risk taking, creativity in adversity) could be subsumed under these three rubrics. "Hardiness" seems to describe a constellation of personality traits that keeps people physically well under stress and psychologically well facing a life crisis such as illness.

The concept of hardiness proposed by social psychologists overlaps to some degree with the psychoanalytic term *ego strength,* which MacKinnon and Yudofsky (1986) defined as the effectiveness of all ego functions in promoting the adaptation of the organism to the environment. They suggested that ego strength depends on "the quality and stability of the emotional ties to others, on the elastic adaptation to instinctual demands and on optimal freedom from the reactive affects of anxiety and guilt" (p. 235). For several reasons, I find the term incomplete in describing the kind of courage and optimism my patients demonstrated. First, despite the efforts of investigators like Cooper et al. (1966), the concept of ego strength remains vague and elusive. Second, assessments of ego functioning or ego strength tend to focus on the unconscious mental processes involved in psychological adaptation (like defenses) and leave out the largely conscious cognitive-behavioral strategies so important to patients' coping. Psychoanalytic inquiry, on the other hand, offers a longitudinal perspective on the vicissitudes of coping and is concerned with the psychogenesis of adult behavior that cognitive psychologists tend to ignore.

Following Anthony (1987), I propose the term *resilience* as an initial and tentative attempt to bridge the gap between these differing viewpoints. In trying to describe and understand how some individuals withstand and rebound so well from adversity, I felt we needed a psychodynamic and psychogenetic perspective on this phenomenon, which the analysts have called "ego strength," coupled with the cognitive-social psychologists' understanding of that particular way of seeing oneself and the world called "hardiness."

Psychoanalytic thinkers have used the intensive study of individual cases as a way of trying to understand and delineate the earliest origins of resilience. In a questionnaire study of psychological responses to colectomy that I undertook in 1969, I observed (as Cousins did) that patients tended to be divided into two groups: those who adjusted well to the colostomy viewed it as a challenge to be mastered, whereas those who adjusted poorly regarded it as a wound deserving of recompense. In Chapter 1, I suggested that the crucial element distinguishing the two groups is the deep, unconscious sense of betrayal that plagues patients in the latter group. Patients who do badly are full of blame and recrimination.

In contrast, the three individuals whose stories I presented here did not ask "Why me?" and did not look to blame others when faced with infirmity. Their stories suggest that there were at least three sources for this healthy view of the self and sense of assurance in the face of physical ailment. First, they had as role models and figures for identification parents who advocated robustness, exuberance, and self-reliance and applauded these qualities in their children. Second, previous experience of mastery over infirmity enabled them to confront new challenges with a sense of competence and exhilaration rather than fear and despair. In a sense, their mettle had already been tested and proved sound.

A third source of strength in these three individuals requires a bit more explanation. Anthony (1987) addressed personality characteristics that "insulate" an individual from future adverse life experiences and bestow an apparent "psychoimmunity" to the effects of deprivation. He postulated that some children have a "buffering system" composed of such factors as stimulus barriers against undue excitation, have adequate maternal empathy and caretaking, and have an "inoculation" effect of certain early challenges against later stressful events. The major focus is the "ego and its acquired mechanisms of resilience," and Anthony emphasized ego resources such as problem solving, ability to make meaningful sense out of chaotic external events, and interpersonal skills, among others. Also, as in my first proposition, he found that "good copers" seemed to have parents who were models of resilience, and he stressed identification with a resilient caregiver.

Treatment Implications

What are the implications of these observations for the care of patients such as those I have described? Unlike some patients who gladly yield control and passively place themselves in the hands of their physicians, these individuals often insist on taking a very active role in their treatment and require a sense of partnership with their doctors. Their care can be time consuming because each demands to be viewed as a special case, an exception to the statistical rules. If the available data have yielded a single clear prescription for the care of these patients, it is that their belief in a positive outcome and in their ability to influence that outcome should be supported and not challenged. Psychiatric consultation is generally neither sought nor required. When such consultation is necessary, extraordinary flexibility is required by the psychiatrist, who cannot be wedded to one technique or modality. Often, working with the primary physician or the patient's family may be all that is necessary or desirable. For other patients, a cognitive-behavioral approach may bolster formerly successful but flagging modes of adaptation. With these patients, the therapist should be prepared to oscillate between giving permission to express loss and anger at the illness and maintaining optimism and hope. The therapist must remain sufficiently removed from the medical or surgical team so that he or she can operate in both these roles. Patients' responses to the therapist's hopefulness will be a transference repetition of the response they had originally to the sanguine parent. For a selective few patients, the crisis of illness may provide an entry into the patient's ongoing life, and psychodynamic psychotherapy offers a dramatic opportunity for a reevaluation of life goals. Either way, these remain interesting, productive, and highly challenging patients whose courage, optimism, and resilience can be an inspiration to those of us entrusted with their care.

References

Anthony EJ: Risk invulnerability and resilience: an overview, in The Invulnerable Child. Edited by Anthony EJ, Cohler BJ. New York, Guilford, 1987, pp 3–49

Beisser AR: Denial and affirmation in illness and health. Am J Psychiatry 136:1026–1030, 1979

Breznitz S: The Denial of Stress. New York, International Universities Press, 1983, pp 257–280

Cooper AM, Karush A, Easser BR, et al: The adaptive balance profile and prediction of early treatment behavior, in Developments in Psychoanalysis at Columbia. Edited by Goldman G, Shapiro D. New York, Hafner, 1966, pp 183–214

Cousins N: Anatomy of an Illness as Perceived by the Patient. New York, Bantam, 1979, pp 49–70

Cousins N: The Healing Heart. New York, WW Norton, 1983

Dean C, Surtees P: Do psychologic factors predict survival in breast cancer? J Psychosom Res 33:561–589, 1989

Druss RG, O'Connor JF, Stern LO: Psychologic response to colectomy, II: adjustment to a permanent colostomy. Arch Gen Psychiatry 20:419–427, 1969

Dubos R: Introduction, in Anatomy of an Illness as Perceived by the Patient. By Cousins N. New York, Bantam, 1979, pp 11–23

Fareed O: Afterwards, in The Healing Heart. By Cousins N. New York, WW Norton, 1983, pp 249–275

Folks D, Freeman A, Sokol M, et al: Denial: predictor of outcome following coronary bypass surgery. Int J Psychiatry Med 18:57–66, 1988

Hackett TP, Cassem NH: Development of a quantitative rating scale to assess denial. J Psychosom Res 18:93–100, 1974

Kobasa SC, Maddi SR, Kahn S: Hardiness and health: a prospective study. J Pers Soc Psychol 42:168–177, 1982

Kobasa SC, Ouellette K, Puccetti MC: Personality and social resources in stress resistance. J Pers Soc Psychol 45:839–850, 1983

Lazarus RS: The costs and benefits of denial, in The Denial of Stress. Edited by Breznitz S. New York, International Universities Press, 1983, pp 1–30

Levinson J, Mishra A, Hamer RM, et al: Denial and medical outcome in unstable angina. Psychosom Med 51:27–35, 1989

Levy S, Lee J, Bagley C, et al: Survival hazards in first recurrent breast cancer patients: seven-year follow-up. Psychosom Med 50:520–528, 1988

Locke SE: Stress, adaptation and immunity: studies in humans. Gen Hosp Psychiatry 4:49–58, 1982

MacKinnon RA, Yudofsky SC: The Psychiatric Evaluation in Clinical Practice. Philadelphia, PA, JB Lippincott, 1986

Perry S, Viederman M: Management of emotional reactions to acute medical illness. Med Clin North Am 65:3–14, 1981

Peterson C, Seligman M, Vaillant G: Pessimistic explanatory style is a risk factor for physical illness: a thirty-five-year longitudinal study. J Pers Soc Psychol 55:23–27, 1988

Pettingale KW, Philalithis A, Tee DEH, et al: The biologic correlates of psychological responses to breast cancer. J Psychosom Res 25:453–458, 1981

Scheier MF, Carver CS: Dispositional optimism and physical well-being: the influence of generalized outcome expectations on health. J Pers 55:169–210, 1987

60 Minutes, Vol 13, No 36, as broadcast over CBS Television Network, Sunday, May 24, 1981

7

Courage Facing
Chronic Illness

With Special Reference to the Life of
Robert Louis Stevenson

Courage falls within the domain of psychiatry. Everyone's life contains experiences ranging from the difficult to the dreadful that either bring people into psychotherapy or arise during its course. Our patients are sorely tested all the time by the "thousand natural shocks that flesh is heir to" (*Hamlet*, III:1).

Yet, despite offering the most elegant exposition on the origins and the vicissitudes of anxiety, psychoanalysis has had little to say about courage. In both of Freud's theories of anxiety, he used concepts of danger and trauma and loss and conflict; his psychoanalytic followers have for the most part continued to use these models.

Other disciplines have also focused their attention on anxiety. Neurophysiologists describe the somatic components of anxiety employing such concepts as fight-flight responses, emergency emotions, and aversive conditioning. Animals have been shocked and humans intubated searching for the deeper effects of anxiety on the organism.

More recently, three additional disciplines have added to our understanding of anxiety. Child observers (Emde and Harmon 1984; Stern 1985) have demonstrated that the earliest interactions between mother and child will lead to a setting that can provide either safety or fear and that those individuals who receive the message that the world is dangerous will walk the world in fear the rest of their lives. They have found that phobic parents produce phobic offspring. The neonatologists take it back even further and see a difference at birth (or even in utero) in the degree of neuromuscular irritability. They can predict, I believe, with some accuracy who will be phlegmatic and who will become a bundle of nerves come 20 years later. Physiology, not anatomy, is destiny. And, finally, there have been the exciting studies on neurotransmitters and fear (Klein 1987); various natural chemicals protect against the anxious state, and receptor sites must be attached lest the person become fearful. Some studies have focused on panic attacks (Gorman 1987), anxiety in its extreme form, and the pharmacological treatment of this disorder. Providing a substance missing to a panic-prone individual is similar to giving insulin to someone with diabetes; it appears that fear is a deficiency disease.

I believe we should approach the subject of courage from a somewhat different vantage point. As a psychoanalyst working with patients with serious and chronic medical illness, I have of course seen anxiety, but so too have I seen unexplained courage. I have treated those who were overcome as much by the fear of their illness as by the illness itself and those who have somehow been able to rise above it. The facts and realities were not different, but some patients faced them with optimism and acceptance. It is not only the absence of fear but the addition of some other quality—courage—that is different in these individuals' responses; this chapter is an exploration of that quality.

The totality of any human being's life is greater than the sum of its parts. We can spend many fruitful hours analyzing even the simplest Bach fugue, understand the organization, the flow of its themes, the reversals and alternations used by the composer—but it will never equal the beauty of a performance. We can obtain the recipe for the famous crème brûlée served to the happy patrons at the Lutèce restaurant, but a list of its ingredients does not remotely portend the few minutes of its exquisite taste. This is not a diatribe against analysis of music or literature or a Lutèce dessert, because such study adds to our appreciation; we just should not be fooled that the fugue, poem, or food is only the sum of its ingredients. Any examination of human beings requires a dissection into their components to make a start in understanding them—but we are more than a collection of drives or a bag of enzymes.

Traditional psychoanalysis has had a particular problem with virtue. Being reductionistic, it tries to explain the positive emotions or virtues in terms of the two libidinal drives of sex and aggression. Courage, self-sacrifice, and altruism and all other positive feelings are to be derived from these two basic drives. Bravery in rescuing a stranger from a burning building could be seen ultimately as reaction formation against fear or an atonement for the guilt of past sins. Bravery in defense of a spouse or a parent or even country could be seen as a drive derivative in which the erotic component remains unconscious. I don't think classical psychoanalysis has ever really come to grips with the virtues beyond such Euclidean attempts to derive all behavior from the fewest basic axioms.

Gaylin (1973), in his essay "Skinner Redux," has similar criticisms to make about the behaviorism of B. F. Skinner. He feels that behaviorism finds any piece of behavior ultimately comprehensible as the complex end point of experience and conditioning. Psychic determinism is central to behaviorism and allows no place for free choice or free action. If all acts are compelled, there is no place for any "virtue," including courage. Humankind's experience includes more than the sum of small learnings.

As a first way out of this reductionism, Gaylin emphasized the concept of identification, in which the life experience of another person can be taken en bloc without having to go through one's own personal experience: "Whole modes of behavior will be instituted by that strange mechanism halfway to love that we call identification" (p. 54). Courage involves the process of identification with a brave parent.

A second concept that has been introduced more recently into psychoanalysis is ego strength—how effectively an individual adapts to his or her own environment. (I described ego strength in greater detail in Chapter 6, "Healthy Denial.") Clearly, ego strength and mastery will have an intimate relationship to courage.

An additional important contribution to modern psychoanalytic thinking is outlined by Kohut (1985) in his concept of "the nuclear self," discussed in his posthumously published essay, "On Courage." He felt that "among those selves there is one most centrally located in the psyche: the nuclear self. It is composed of derivatives of the grandiose self of goal and ambition, and derivatives of the idealized parent imago; it contains our most enduring values and ideals" (pp. 10–11). He further stated that courage cannot be explained only as the personification and concretization of the ego ideal. The hero is compelled to "proceed on his lonely road, even if it means his individual destruction, because he must shape his life in accordance with the design of that 'nuclear self'" (p. 9).

Another way in which we can escape the inherent reductionism of both classical psychoanalysis and classical behaviorism is by turning to evolution and thinking about the place of humans in the animal kingdom. There may well be a survival value placed on courage that is part of the genetic history of humankind. Thomas (1983) described altruism as one of biology's deep mysteries. Why should an animal choose to give up its life to to aid another? At first glance, it seems an unnatural act, even a violation of nature. A worker bee patrolling the hive who senses a stranger will sting it, an act of self-sacrifice because stinging kills the bee. Thomas continued that many higher animals manifest altruistic behavior. A male bird will attract the attention of a predator to protect a nest of fledglings. Why is this so? What happened to survival of the fittest? Thomas feels that the *unit* of survival is the species, not the individual. The genes must be preserved, not any given carrier of them. Also, humans are by nature social animals, not solitary animals, with all the ethological cues toward social behaviors. So we come by our bravery honestly. Inclinations toward altruism, in and of itself, exist in all of us and need not be reducible to some other drive, which is to say courage may not always be noble, but it is not simply a defense against cowardice.

There is perhaps an additional reason why psychiatry has taken such a scanty view of the virtues. Growing out of medicine, psychiatry is grounded in pathology and dysfunction. The physician is trained to look at what is wrong or aberrant or a departure from healthy functioning. Only now have views such as "wellness" and "holistic medicine" come into vogue. Yet they have early historical origins outside of medicine and science.

Perhaps one might now turn from the natural sciences to natural philosophy to get a new perspective on an age-old problem. What is courage, and where does it come from?

First, a few definitions. *Courage* is the quality of mind or spirit that enables one to face difficulty, danger, and pain (*bravery* implies boldness and daring in action as well). In any discussion of courage, one has to rule out bravado, impulsivity, and denial.

The ignorant man who does not even know he is facing danger cannot be considered brave, just foolish. Bravery requires full knowledge of all the rules, and action occurs despite that knowledge. The behavior must be sensible.

The man who is drunk or hallucinating or infantile and has poor impulse control cannot be considered brave. He is foolhardy and acts without reason.

Then there is the question of denial. *Pathological denial* is a mechanism of defense whereby unpleasant or frightening realities are kept out of consciousness. This is a pathological response, however, and also cannot be seen as courageous.

So, we regard the courageous human as one who has full knowledge of the danger; there must also be a reasonableness to his or her acts. Courage facing chronic illness seems to require 1) endurance, 2) readiness for action, and 3) the ability to make optimistic choices.

Elements of Courage Facing Chronic Illness

Endurance

Endurance is surely the cornerstone of courage. Plato would seem to be the logical place to begin an exploration of endurance. Each of the early so-called Socratic dialogues by Plato is concerned with a different virtue or excellence: the *Charmides* with temperance, the *Lysis* with friendship, the *Euthyphro* with piety, etc. The *Laches* discusses courage. The dialogue begins with the various participants discussing the value of gymnastics, martial arts, and war games as preparation for courage in battle. But Socrates asked them what is the common element in all forms of courage, not only in battle but also when facing perils by sea and natural disaster, poverty, disease, and pain. He arrives at the conclusion that this common element is endurance.

The Stoic philosophers valued an acceptance of life and harmony with nature. They declared it to be humans' duty to obey the divine law of their reason, which can raise them above the troubles of daily life and provide courage when facing illness, old age, and death.

Marcus Aurelius is steeped in the stoical tradition. He concluded in his "Meditations" that true courage starts with acceptance and duty, which over a lifetime leads to endurance. Epictetus, the great Stoic philosopher and mentor of Marcus Aurelius, stated that "the path to contentment was to dispossess yourself in advance of all that was out of your power—then fortunes shocks might rain down unfelt" (quoted in James 1908). Endurance is the common end point for both Plato and the Stoics.

My experience with seriously ill people has demonstrated that the surest way out of self-absorption and self-pity is through the performance of one's duty. Alcoholics Anonymous discovered long ago that endurance involves taking "each day one at a time" and going about one's business.

What is the intrapsychic experience of a man or woman who is enduring a serious chronic illness?

1. It involves some renunciation of expectations of the perfect life and the acceptance of what life has to offer. William James (1908) elaborated on this point: "I, who for the time have staked my all on being a psychologist, am mortified when others know much more psychology than I. But I am contented to wallow in the grossest ignorance of Greek. My deficiencies there give me no sense of personal humiliation at all. To give up pretensions is as blessed a relief as to get them gratified! There is a lightness about the heart when one's nothingness in a particular line is accepted in good faith" (p. 310).
2. The boundaries of the self are shrunk and the illness viewed as external to one's essence rather than as a part of it. One reduces one's boundaries to Kohut's (1985) "nuclear self."
3. There is a turning within to fantasy and imagination as the external world temporarily or periodically is allowed to fade. I elaborate on this point later in this chapter, when discussing Stevenson.
4. There must be a self-soothing mechanism available that can be called on when needed; I feel this is laid down very early. One thinks of little Jessica McClure, age 18 months, trapped at the bottom of a well. The public was gripped by the story and her eventual 58-hour rescue. During the ordeal, she was heard singing to herself and giving herself a musical pep talk.

Action

Courage is more than endurance. One can turn the other cheek only so far before one's head is facing backward. The second element involves risk taking and action. It consists of a challenge, and a challenge overcome. Aristotle comes to the virtues from a different starting point than does Plato. In the "Nichomachean Ethics," Aristotle stated that humans become builders by building and lyre players by playing the lyre. Like skills, we acquire virtues by exercising them. In our transactions with others, we become just or unjust, and in our acts accomplished in the presence of danger, we become brave or cowardly. Courage, he stated, is therefore a habit of the soul.

In a recent study, B. Druss (1985) investigated the motivation of winners of the Carnegie Hero Award, which is given annually to 100 private citizens who risk their lives to save others from personal injury or death such as from a fire or drowning. The conclusion was that such behavior was not related to moral choice but rather to extensive prior exposure to dangerous situations and previous mastery of them.

In Chapter 6, "Healthy Denial," I described adaptive responses to illness and disability. The individuals described in that chapter did not disavow the fact of their particular infirmity. They "preferred" to evaluate the situation from the most favorable viewpoint and believed that they could beat the odds. They felt they could positively influence the course of their illness or disability and overcome the challenge. They were remarkably free of narcissism and of self-pity and envy toward others. A common thread was the presence of parental role models and figures for identification who advocated robustness and applauded these qualities in their children from an early age. In addition, previous experience of mastery over infirmity enabled them to confront new challenges with a sense of competence and exhilaration. I used the term *resiliency* to describe this combination of hardiness and ego strength.

All these characteristics involve activity versus passivity, risk taking, and creative solutions to new problems as they arrive. Individuals who possess these qualities see today's glass as half full rather than half empty and see tomorrow's that way as well. Action is now to be added to endurance. There is a dynamic tension between these two attributes: When should one act to fight against the chronic disease, and when should one endure it, accept the limitations the disease imposes, and make peace with them? This is the most crucial and most basic dilemma that faces chronically ill people.

For the individual faced with chronic illness, there is a constant need to make such a choice. When should one get another opinion, try some experimental yet unproven remedy, undergo a risky surgical procedure or intervention *(action)*? Or, when should one make peace with one's disability and try to derive as much pleasure from life as one can, despite the disability *(endurance)*? There is never a final answer: symptoms worsen or new drugs arrive on the scene that require one to shift from the stoical position to one more action oriented. (Not to make this shift would be a manifestation of passivity rather than endurance.) At its best, courage involves a flexible and fluid shift between endurance and action.

Optimistic Choice

The final component of courage is that of choice. First we must understand that choice *is* a possibility. Modern physics, which underlies modern biology, is a physics of unpredictability. Heisenberg's "uncertainty principle" states that one does not have the ability to predict the action and location of any given electron; particle physicists may know the rate of radioactive decay but not which atom will be the next to decay.

Gleick, in his fascinating new book *Chaos: Making a New Science* (1988), discussed the randomness and unpredictability in the physical world. He devoted one chapter, "Inner Rhythms," to biological phenomena. He cited Edwin Schrödinger, the quantum physicist, who had an interest in biological speculation: "Schrödinger felt that the building block of life was an aperiodic crystal (today's DNA). To see aperiodicity as the source of life's special quality verged on the mystical. Pattern born amid formlessness: that is biology's basic beauty, and its basic mystery" (p. 299).

Courage not only involves the possibility of choice but the necessity of choice. At any given point in one's life, one can choose to act optimistically or pessimistically, with bravery or with cowardice. One will not always be true to the task; the circumstances may vary, and one's sense of resoluteness may vary from one day to the next. Optimism about the outcome will influence both one's state of mind and how one acts on any given occasion. It is my contention that people have even more control than they realize over how they feel on any given day. Cognitive therapy suggests that to some extent optimism can be learned (Beck and Freeman 1990).

The genetic and constitutional theories of anxiety clearly state that humans have no choice by the time we are fully formed adults and that we all are prisoners of our makeup. Psychoanalysis has as one of its unstated tenets the axiom of predetermination; we are what we were, and we repeat rather than remember. So what is the individual to do who requires the courage he or she was not born with or did not learn?

Psychoanalysis is a therapy as well as a theory. As a therapy, it is based on an equally strong belief that change in adult life *is* possible. The potential for alteration may be limited, but small alterations may offer the possibility of big change. Psychoanalysis and psychodynamic psychotherapy can help people expand their options and increase the opportunities for self-mastery and a sense of mastery of their circumstances. The neurotic underpinnings of anxiety can be exposed and often eliminated. The symbolic meaning of any disease or disorder can be understood in the light of each individual's uniqueness and past experience. The special techniques and modifications of psychodynamic psychotherapy with medical patients were discussed in Chapter 5, "Treatment Philosophy." Surely the optimistic and life-affirming attitude of the therapist will help those patients who from time to time cannot call on these resources within themselves.

I would like to illustrate many of the theoretical points made so far by an example, the life of Robert Louis Stevenson.

The Life of Robert Louis Stevenson

The information I have about the life of Robert Louis Stevenson is taken from a biography by Daiches (1973), two biographical sketches by Kiely (1983) and Boyle (1987), an article by Greenacre (1978) discussing Stevenson's dispute with William Henley, the introduction to *The Strange Case of Dr. Jekyll and Mr. Hyde* by Stevenson's wife Fanny V. deG. Stevenson, an essay by Steinberg (1951), and the nonfictional writings of Stevenson himself. I concentrate on his lifelong illness, which was the organizing principle of his life, and leave to the reader to discover on his or her own the interesting matters regarding his relationships with women and the discussions of his popular fictional output.

Robert Louis Balfour Stevenson was born on November 13, 1850, in Edinburgh. He was the only child of Thomas Stevenson and Margaret Balfour. Thomas was a lighthouse engineer; the Stevensons were a prosperous Victorian family.

For our purposes, the most important thing to say about Louis, as he was called, was that he was sickly from the day of his birth. He had almost continuous respiratory infections in his infancy, which progressed to pulmonary tuberculosis in childhood, and he was at death's door for virtually all his life. He wrote as an adult, "I have not had a day's real health; I have awakened sick and gone to bed weary. I have written in bed and written out of it, written in hemorrhages, written in sickness, written torn by coughing, written when my head swam for weakness; for so long it seems to me I have won my wager and recovered my glove." (quoted in Steinberg, p. 296).

According to his biographers, his mother was distant and uninvolved. Alice Cunningham came to look after Louis when he was 18 months old. He shared a room with "Cummy," as he called her, until he was 10. Cummy played the positive maternal role in Louis's life, and they were very close. She tended him when he was in the throes of his frequent childhood ailments with great devotion and imagination. He never forgot her, and when he grew up he dedicated *A Child's Garden of Verses* (1885), a collection of poems based on his own vivid childhood memories, to her:

> For the long nights you lay awake
> And watched for my unworthy sake.
> For your most comfortable hand,
> That led me through the uneven land . . .
> My second Mother, my first Wife,
> The angel of my infant life.

He wrote later about his early years of sickness when he would lay awake at night praying for sleep or for morning to come. He described the devotion of his father, who came to his bedside filled with exciting stories to distract Louis during his paroxysms. Louis's father had a lively imagination and would tell stories of "ships, roadside inns, robbers, sailors, and travelers before the era of steam" (Daiches 1973, p. 8). His father encouraged Louis when Louis began to create his first tales of romantic adventure.

Stevenson attended Edinburgh University and then law school. He never practiced law, preferring the literary life, where his talents lay. In 1880, he married Fanny Osborn. Fanny was more than 10 years older than Louis. She remained at his side throughout all his travels and was as much a nurse as a wife. Surely, the prototype of Fanny was Cummy, the nurse of his infancy.

Stevenson traveled often, primarily to find a climate and locale that would be kind to his ailments. He lived for a time in Monterey, California, and San Francisco. Trips to Scotland from time to time were unbearable due to the hostile climate, and he traveled instead to the city of Davos in Switzerland, the scene of Thomas Mann's *The Magic Mountain*. Stevenson sought and received the best medical attention available to him at the time.

In 1888, Stevenson set out from San Francisco to the South Pacific, where he remained the rest of his life. The tropics were the only place where he did not experience repeated respiratory infections. He settled in Samoa, an exile from his beloved Scotland and many friends, and died in 1894.

Stevenson manifested all the qualities of courage discussed previously. His endurance and "stick-to-itiveness" were legendary in his lifetime. He was a popular author; his collected works number 32 volumes, including *Treasure Island* and *Kidnapped*. He had the ability to enter the world of fantasy, re-creating that bond with a loving, approving father. The benign regression when the illness was in exacerbation took him into an inner world of creative imagination where he could become like his early, storytelling father. Furthermore, Stevenson had the capacity to work through the apprehensions about his disease in his writings. One example of this is his depiction of the character Long John Silver, the one-legged pirate of *Treasure Island*. The character was modeled after his former friend and rival William Henley, who was an amputee secondary to tuberculosis that had lodged in his bone. Greenacre (1978) feels that the horror Louis must have experienced seeing this gruesome effect of tuberculosis was externalized in the book. It is an example of Stevenson's use of his creativity to contain primitive fears of mutilation.

A second example of coping with early anxiety by mastering it in his creative output was described by Fanny Stevenson. She said that there was a chest of drawers in his nursery made by the notorious Deacon Brodie— the respectable craftsman by day and burglar by night. Apparently, Cummy wove many stories about mundane objects of furniture in his room to distract young Louis; some were apparently quite lurid. The latent memories of Deacon Brodie gave the germ of an idea that developed into the short story "Markheim" and, finally, in a hectic fever following a hemorrhage of the lungs, culminated in the dream of Dr. Jekyll and Mr. Hyde. Fanny described how Louis was usually a very sound sleeper, but one night she awoke him from a fitful sleep, and he went immediately to his pad and scribbled a rapid outline of *The Strange Case of Dr. Jekyll and Mr. Hyde*. At daybreak in the midst of a high fever, he began the new book. In 3 days, the first draft of

32,000 words was furiously written; it was ready for press by 3 weeks. At this time, she stated, Louis was so infirm he could barely speak, and conversation was by slate and pencil. His visitors were limited to 15 minutes, with Fanny standing guard at the door. She felt that he wrote his best when he was sickest and febrile and admired his courage in doing so.

Yet Stevenson was a man of action. He showed the willingness to move throughout the globe to locate the most salubrious climate. He demanded and received the best medical care available in his lifetime. In 1887–1888, during that harsh winter, Stevenson consulted Dr. Edward Trudeau, a famous phthisiologist, in Saranac Lake, New York, who found tuberculosis bacilli in Stevenson's sputum. Trudeau outlined Stevenson's treatment program.

Stevenson was also a vigorous champion of the oppressed. While in Samoa he read of a denunciation of Father Damien of Molokai, Hawaii, the Catholic missionary who tended the large leprosarium there. This provoked fury in Stevenson, who defended Father Damien and attacked the author for his hypocritical sanctimony. Stevenson thought he would be sued for libel and financially ruined, but his considerable anxiety did not deter him from publishing this stinging pamphlet in England. This act required much courage.

Stevenson was a popular man as well as a popular, successful author, and from early on he showed character traits of flexibility, enormous generosity, and friendliness. Few writers inspired such affection in their contemporaries and in later generations of readers. It is difficult to resist the enchanting personality that emerges from his letters. He was a pragmatic Scotsman with the optimism and cheerfulness of the romantic—what Stevenson's biographer Daiches (1973, p. 112) called "endurance combined with a relish for experience."

So, it is interesting that Stevenson, this sickly man, could have written his many adventure stories. It is more interesting that he is the author of "Aes Triplex," considered by many to be the great modern essay on courage. I end the chapter with a generous quote from that essay:

> For surely the love of living is stronger in the Alpine climber roping over a peril, or a hunter riding merrily at a stiff fence, than in a creature who lives upon a diet and walks a measured distance in the interest of his constitution . . . there is but one conclusion possible; that a man should stop his ears

against paralyzing terror, and run the race that is set before him with a single mind. . . . As courage and intelligence are the two qualities best worth a good man's cultivation, so it is the first part of intelligence to recognize our precarious estate in life, and the first part of courage to be not at all abashed before the fact. . . . There is nothing so cruel as panic; the man who has the least fear for his own carcass has the most time to consider others. . . . So soon as prudence has begun to grow up in the brain, like a dismal fungus, it finds its first expression in a paralysis of generous acts . . . for the plain satisfaction of living, of being about their business of some sort or other, do the brave, serviceable men of every nation tread down the nettle danger, and pass flyingly over the stumbling blocks of prudence. . . . Who would find heart enough to begin to live if he dallied with the consideration of death? It is better to lose health like a spendthrift than to waste it like a miser. It is better to live and be done with it than to die daily in the sickroom. By all means begin your folio, even if the doctor does not give you a year, even if he hesitates about a month, make one brave push and see what can be accomplished in a week. Every heart that has beat strong and cheerfully has left a hopeful impulse behind it in the world, and bettered the tradition of mankind. The noise of the mallet and chisel is scarcely quenched, the trumpets are hardly done blowing, when, trailing with him clouds of glory, this happy-starred, full-blooded spirit shoots into the spiritual land. (Stevenson 1903, pp. 108–113)

References

Aristotle: The Nichomachean ethics: book II, in The Basic Works of Aristotle. Edited by McKeon R. New York, Random House, 1941, pp 928–1112

Beck A, Freeman A: Cognitive Therapy of Personality Disorders. New York, Guilford, 1990

Boyle RA: Robert Louis Stevenson, in Dictionary of Literary Biography, Vol 57. Edited by Thesing WB. Detroit, MI, Gail Research, 1987, pp 294–305

Daiches D: Robert Louis Stevenson and His World. London, Thames & Hudson, 1973

Druss B: Carnegie Medal Winners for Heroism. Unpublished senior thesis, Department of Psychology, Swarthmore College, Swarthmore, PA, 1985

Emde R, Harmon R: Entering a new era in the search for developmental continuities, in Continuities and Discontinuities in Development. Edited by Emde R, Harmon R. New York, Plenum, 1984, pp 1–11

Gaylin W: Skinner redux. Harper's Magazine 247:48–56, 1973

Gleick J: Chaos: Making a New Science. New York, Penguin Books, 1988, pp 275–300

Gorman J: Panic disorders, in Anxiety. Edited by Klein D. New York, Karger, 1987, pp 36–91

Greenacre P: Notes on plagiarism: the Henley-Stevenson quarrel. J Am Psychoanal Assoc 26:507–539, 1978

James W: Principles of Psychology, Vol 1. New York, Henry Holt, 1908, pp 309–312

Kiely R: Robert Louis Stevenson, in Dictionary of Literary Biography, Vol 18. Edited by Nadel IB, Fredman W. Detroit, MI, Gail Research, 1983, pp 281–297

Klein D: Anxiety reconceptualized, in Anxiety. Edited by Klein D. New York, Karger, 1987, pp 1–35

Kohut H: On courage, in Self-Psychology and the Humanities: Reflections on a New Psychoanalytic Approach. New York, WW Norton, 1985, pp 3–50

Mann T: The Magic Mountain. New York, Alfred A Knopf, 1955

Marcus Aurelius: The Meditations of Marcus Aurelius. Mount Vernon, NY, Peter Pauper Press, 1942

Plato: The Laches, in The Dialogues of Plato. Translated by Jowett B. New York, Random House, 1937, pp 55–77

Steinberg M: The fear of life, in A Believing Jew. Edited by Steinberg E. New York, Harcourt Brace, 1951, pp 290–300

Stern D: Interpersonal World of the Infant: A View From Psychoanalysis and Developmental Psychology. New York, Basic Books, 1985, pp 188–192

Stevenson FV deG: Introduction, in The Strange Case of Dr. Jekyll and Mr. Hyde. By Stevenson RL. New York, Grolier, 1936, pp i–vii

Stevenson RL: Treasure Island. London, Cassell, 1883

Stevenson RL: A Child's Garden of Verses. London, Longmans, Green, 1885

Stevenson RL: The Strange Case of Dr. Jekyll and Mr. Hyde. London, Longmans, 1886

Stevenson RL: Kidnapped. London, Cassell, 1886

Stevenson RL: Aes triplex, in Virginibus Puerisque and Other Papers. London, Chatto & Windus, 1903, pp 103–113

Thomas L: Altruism, in Late Night Thoughts on Listening to Mahler's Ninth Symphony. New York, Viking, 1983, pp 101–107

8

Exercise, Well-Being, and Restoration

As one walks along the streets and parks of our great cities, the biggest danger to life and limb is not being assaulted by muggers and felons, but being pummeled by the hoards of runners and joggers abounding everywhere. Their ears are encased by Walkmen and their eyes blinded by sweat, oblivious to all others about them. Their cousins can be found in gymnasiums and health clubs, furiously pedaling on their stationary bicycles, or pumping iron. The fitness craze is a new phenomenon and is the confluence of a number of factors.

First, we have a whole class of educated business and professional people who lead enforced sedentary lives. Many hours are spent at the desk or computer, and they crave physical activity. Stevedores don't jog.

Second, as Christopher Lasch (1978) so accurately portrayed it, we live in the age of narcissism. A major component of this age is the desire to look young and fit, the quest for eternal youth and a slim body. These times could also be called the "Diet-Pepsi Generation," with its own emphasis on vitamins, oat bran, and low-calorie drinks.

Sports and physical activity are also a form of play in an ever-increasing workaholic world. Play addresses itself to the child in all of us, moribund but ready to be awakened. Csikszentmihalyi (1990), in his book *Flow*, described the pleasures of play, in which life's problems disappear as one is absorbed fully in activity. In his research, Csikszentmihalyi realized that to induce flow, an individual must be challenged in an activity to the outer limits of his or her capabilities but not beyond them. Exercise is the perfect vehicle for inducement of flow.

Currently, exercise has its "fad" component, and some adherents will drop it next year as they did the Hula Hoop years ago. But exercise is different in a crucial way; exercise is a form of play that has been legitimized by the medical community, supported by a truly vast literature about its health benefits. It has been regarded as the medicine supreme, without side effects, good for reducing the waistline as well as the blood pressure.

The "reversal program" for coronary artery disease developed by Ornish (1990) became the first nonsurgical, nonpharmacological therapy to gain parity with standard and familiar techniques. This program, which involves regular exercise as well as diet, meditation, and support groups, is the first "alternative medical technique" for cardiovascular disease to be reimbursed by a major insurance carrier (Mutual of Omaha Insurance Company). Ornish's "reversal plan," according to the *New York Times* (O'Neill 1993), costs $3,500 per year, which it estimated is about one-tenth the price of conventional coronary care.

In this chapter, I first describe some of the studies that demonstrate the proven value of exercise and being fit as a remedy for both physical and mental illness. Then, I discuss three phenomena that relate exercise and fitness to what I have discussed before: 1) exercise as an inducer of a transcendental mental state, 2) exercise as a treatment for individuals with bodily defects, and 3) restoration of the self and well-being.

Research has demonstrated the value of exercise in reducing the risk for a large variety of illnesses. In 1987, Holmes and Cappo demonstrated the value of exercise in people with type A personalities who were vulnerable to hypertension due to family history. The antihypertensive effects of regular exercise were confirmed more recently by Dunbar (1992). These works are part of a growing literature demonstrating that exercise reduces cardiovascular reactivity to stress. In 1984, Paffenbarger et al. linked exercise to reduced risk for heart attack. In 1983, Krolner et al. demonstrated the value of exercise in reducing bone loss in osteoporosis in elderly people. In 1985, Zinman and Vranic discussed the benefits of regular exercise for people with mild diabetes.

But it was the monumental 1989 study by Blair et al., published in the *Journal of the American Medical Association,* that was most convincing to the public. In this study, 13,000 men and women were followed for 8 years, and those who were most fit had only one-third the death rate from all causes, including heart attack, than did the least fit. Most comforting was the finding that the correlation was linear, with some benefits derived from any degree of exercise—walking was almost as good as running, and something better than nothing. These findings made the daily papers and network television news and opened an avenue to the multitudes who knew they could never spend an hour a day training for the triathlon. Exercise was no longer just for athletes and ex-athletes but a potential blessing for everyone.

There are additional studies that deal with exercise as therapeutic for mental health. In a controlled study, Ossip-Klein et al. (1989) investigated 40 clinically depressed women and noted significant improvements in mood and self-concept in those assigned to a running program. These improvements were maintained over time as long as the running was continued. Schwartz (1989) noted exercise intolerance and poor cardiovascular fitness in many anxious patients and felt that there was a negative interpretation of the sympathetic arousal that occurred normally during exercise. He recommended supervised exercise for patients with panic disorder and generalized anxiety as a way of overcoming this problem. Berger and Owen (1987) studied the effects of swimming on anxiety in 100 college students. They found significantly less anxiety in these students after they swam than before, regardless of the exercise duration and intensity. The program was equally as good for reducing cognitive anxiety as it was for reducing somatic anxiety symptoms. Sixty-one sedentary working women were studied by Long (1985) and Long and Haney (1988). Aerobic conditioning through regular jogging resulted in significantly less anxiety and greater self-efficacy in these women. Morgan and Goldston (1987) have written a number of articles on anxiety reduction brought on by vigorous exercise. They found that highly anxious individuals experienced a significant reduction in anxiety following strenuous physical activity.

In 1979, Greist et al. suggested that running was at least as effective as psychotherapy in the treatment of mild to moderate depression. Greist regards running as a nonradical, cost-effective treatment. A runner himself, he conducts some of his sessions running with his depressed patients. In another article, Sacks (1984) discussed the uses of exercise from a psychodynamic point of view. He concluded that running is related to the "practicing period" in infancy. When individuals seek to master physical stress in adulthood, they may return to physical solutions such as running rather than to verbal expression, such as thinking or fantasy. Sacks (1990), however, added a cautionary note. The antidepressant effects of exercise last only one day, and therefore one would need to run daily to gain a lasting antidepressant effect. (This is in contrast to the three-times-a-week programs designed for cardiovascular fitness.)

Simons et al. (1985) surveyed the literature on exercise as a treatment for depression. They felt that early research on the mental effects of exercise had many conceptual and methodological problems. They cited more recent studies based on biochemical and physiological variables and concluded that the explanation for improvement in depression is based on the fact that exercise produces specific physiological changes. There is evidence that other effective somatic treatments for depression such as electroconvulsive therapy and tricyclic antidepressants produce changes in aminergic synaptic transmission. Simons et al. feel that exercise-induced improvements in mood may also be due to increased aminergic transmission. The other biochemical approach they discuss attributes the antidepressant effect to increases in beta-endorphin activity, and they quote numerous studies supporting this explanation. Lobstein et al. (1989) pursued the beta-endorphin hypothesis. They compared 10 active middle-aged (40–60 years) men with 10 sedentary men. They concluded that these two groups could be distinguished on the basis of a profile that included a determination of resting plasma beta-endorphin activity.

The most comprehensive review of exercise and sports in mental health was conducted by Glesser and Mendelberg (1990). There was convincing evidence that physical activity had marked benefits on anxiety reduction, mood elevation, and increased self-esteem, and the authors regard it as a practical, inexpensive treatment modality.

Exercise Inducing a Transcendental State

I feel that quite beyond the benefits of reducing anxiety and restoring mood, solo exercise has a quality that is unexplained by such improvement. Running, lap swimming, and stationary-bike riding involve repetition as well as movement and lead to a benign loss of self-awareness. A study of aspiring ballet students attempted to answer the question of what motivated these young women to undertake a program of self-denial and grueling daily practice sessions when they fully realized that the odds were greatly against their achieving stardom or even achieving any position with a ballet company (Druss and Silverman 1979). The anticipation of some future performance was not the major motivation because most of their time was spent in the ritualistic repetitive practice for some possible future event rather than performing in the event itself. The students reported that during practice, they often achieved a state "beyond boredom," a transcendental state with its own special pleasure. Pianists also spend hours practicing scales or doing and redoing a piece countless times. Their fingers are doing the ballerina's compulsory exercises. At times it is a necessary torture, but at least some of the time they also describe a total absorption in the work during which the cares of the world briefly disappear. The vigorous bodily swaying of Orthodox Jews at prayer with the repetition of certain passages again and again may be seen as another example of this phenomenon.

Solomon and Bumpers (1978) describe the running meditation response as a "new" method for inducing a relaxation response that employs both long-distance running and the relaxation response postulated by Benson (1975). They do not see this method as generally applicable to all patients, and its effects vary. But, in some patients, an improvement in well-being can be activated by simultaneous slow running and meditation.

Exercise as a Treatment for Bodily Defects

Two years after a major heart attack, a man in his late 40s came to me for psychotherapy of an intractable low-level depression. He had already tried a year of classical psychoanalysis, with no benefit. He said he had no intention of taking antidepressant medication because he was already taking two cardiac drugs, aspirin and propranolol and hated the idea of being a patient. He had been a fine athlete all his life, proud of his physique and physical prowess. The coronary came as a surprise despite a risky family history and was a narcissistic blow that "hit him where he lived." The advice of his cardiologist to "take it easy" angered him, and the daily concern of his loving wife infuriated him. He had lost all interest in his work, his wife, and his children, and the zest for living that had been his usual mode of adaptation before he was stricken with the coronary was gone. He had no vegetative signs and no suicidal ideation, but when I first saw him he looked like a beaten man, old before his time.

The treatment proceeded well, with the initial therapeutic task being to win his trust and get to know him. He had little aptitude for reflection or introspection. He had a mildly hypomanic, action-prone, type A personality and was used to the idea that he could accomplish what he had set out to do.

After about 6 months, I asked him whether he had tried the special cardiofitness program at the local Y. He had not heard of it and jumped at the idea. He joined and spent many of our sessions describing the program. He derived enormous comfort from being with a group of "walking wounded all in the same boat." They were his kind of people—long on action, short on talk. The physical program involved graduated, carefully monitored sessions on the stationary bicycles and some gentle lap swimming. He kept meticulous charts and graphs of his progress and took great pleasure in the slow but steady rise in the curve. At last—a challenge he could master.

Our treatment lasted 1.5 years. He left without depression and with "a new lease on life." He was grateful that I had listened to his "bitching" and felt that the fitness program I had suggested was the most important ingredient in "our therapy."

This account is typical of many postcoronary patients I have treated in recent years. My interpretations regarding his castration anxiety and resulting sense of deficit were accepted but not usable until put to the acid test— the gym. Taylor et al. (1986) came to the same conclusion in a study of 210 postmyocardial infarction patients. Those in cardiovascular exercise programs improved 3–26 weeks after myocardial infarction on all anxiety and depression measures.

In previous chapters, I suggested that the "talking therapies" alone are often insufficient treatments for patients with physical illness. I have lauded the value of groups like Weight Watchers, physical ministrations like massage and physical therapy, and bedside nursing for those who are in pain or are acutely ill. For many of the patients I see, men and women both, those with coronary disease, hypertension, and obesity, surely, but also those with cured cancer or chronic neurological diseases, exercise is a necessary part of their psychiatric treatment. One can almost make the statement that when a physical defect or limitation is present, words alone will not be enough. The physical sense of the defect must include a physical element in its cure. Such a proposition has too often been characterized as facilitating denial, aiding resistance, or even colluding in acting out.

Freud (1923, p. 26)) said that "the ego is originally a body ego . . . ultimately derived from bodily sensations." What Freud meant was that the infant in the crib, as it exercises its limbs and explores its small world, is at the same time delineating its boundaries and distinguishing self from nonself. People with medical afflictions must go through a similar physical process, also using their muscular and tactile experiences, as they begin the process of rehabilitation. They must physically relearn their abilities and their limitations.

Participation in vigorous exercise is as new as today's fad, as I noted at the start of this chapter. But it is as old as medicine itself, when good diet, fresh air, and exercise were recommended by physicians everywhere. This prescription is typified by Donaldson (1962) in *Strong Medicine,* a delightful book written by a canny practitioner who gave physician and patient alike clear advice about treatment of common chronic illnesses: "To my thinking the greatest advance in recorded medical history is the thirty-minute walk before breakfast. Premiums for life insurance are usually paid for the benefit of someone else. If you want any life insurance for yourself you had better pay the daily premium of a thirty-minute walk" (p. 46). He further noted, "There seems to be nothing that relieves the anxiety state so well as hard outdoor exercise and useful work" (p. 126). Dr. Donaldson was 30 years ahead of his time.

Well-Being and Restoration

I have discussed a number of the significant terms used to describe the salutary state: *hardiness,* used by Kobasa et al. (1983); *ego strength,* used by dynamic psychiatrists and psychoanalysts; and *resiliency,* which I used to try to explain "healthy denial" (although the term was used in a somewhat different manner by Beardslee in 1989).

Each of these terms is useful. But as a dynamic therapist working on a daily basis with patients coping with chronic and awful medical conditions, I still am faced with the question: Where does one acquire hardiness, ego strength, and resilience, and how do we help those people whose coping mechanisms are flagging or overwhelmed achieve some sense of well-being?

I live near one of the avenues where the New York Marathon is run each year. I am not a runner, or a fan of running, so I regard the event as largely a nuisance, what with streets blocked off and all traffic at a standstill for hours. The front-runners pass by at about noon, and the majority of those who will finish pass by at about 3 P.M. But around 5 P.M., when all the police barricades have been taken down, a different group of participants passes by. It is the paraplegics and amputees in their wheelchairs on their way to the finish line. My heart goes out to them, and I often shake their hands as they pass by and receive the firm grip of leather-gloved hands and muscular arms. Are these individuals sick or well? They are disabled, indeed, but they are making a statement to the world and to themselves that they refuse to be counted among the sick.

Emde (1991) wrote that "Freud's concept of motivation was centered around his unpleasure-pleasure principle: unpleasure resulted from increase in drive tension, and pleasure from its decrease. But modern biology has brought us a changed viewpoint . . . *negentropy* characterizes developmental systems" (p. 33). In a brilliant conclusion, he stated, "A good deal of pleasure is linked to negentropy, not entropy. It is exploratory, expectant of novelty, and stimulus seeking. . . . The analyst, through emotional scaffolding, can be thought of as helping to reinstate a capacity for negentropy pleasure in the patient: a capacity for pleasure in experiencing and in integrating what is new" (p. 35).

The common element in all forms of pleasure is that they contribute to an enhanced sense of self, a concept of expansion and creativity. These pleasures involve a reconciliation with our ego-ideal—what we dare hope to be at our best.

Csikszentmihalyi (1990) feels that the ability to take misfortune and make something good come out of it is a great gift. According to him, those who possess this gift are called *survivors* and are said to have "resilience" and "courage." He went on to state the position of the Stoic philosophers that "there are two main strategies we can adopt to improve the quality of life. The first is to try making external conditions match our goals. The second is to change how we experience external conditions to make them better fit our goals" (p. 43). If one does not expect perfect health, security, and happiness and realizes that risks are inevitable, then one can succeed in enjoying a less than ideally predictable world. Csikszentmihalyi especially admires the Stoic philosopher Seneca, who said, "The good things which belong to prosperity are to be wished, but the good things that belong to adversity are to be admired" (p. 200). Of all the virtues we can learn, none is more likely to improve the quality of life than the ability to transform adversity into challenge.

The intrapsychic process of attaining health is through a process of restoration. Baker and Baker (1987) discussed Kohut's self-psychology and indicated that a major focus is on how patients can restore a sense of vitality and harmony to the self when it has been injured by some narcissistic assault.

Courage is a restoration of one's youth. Youth is a time of seeking adventure, taking risks, exploring the world, exercising, and experiencing physical challenge. When one is in the vigor of youth, one feels immortal and that sickness and death are for others.

Well-being is a restoration of one's infancy and early childhood. The infant explores its own immediate world, including its body. If all goes well, the infant exercises, is fed, and sleeps with a depth that adults may envy. We assume it feels omnipotent, the pleasure of primary narcissism—that oceanic pleasure where all is right with the world.

Medically ill people are potentially in a constant state of deprivation and narcissistic injury. Courage alone is not enough. There is a need to help them heal their narcissistic wounds that requires endurance, action, and optimism but that will fail unless we also attend to a repair of the damaged self. Despite illness and physical adversity, that damaged self must be restored, and it is our psychotherapeutic task to help those who cannot do it alone.

The patient thus restored can then say with Horace, *Integer vitae scelerisque purus*—"He who is whole in life need have no fear of the future."

References

Baker HS, Baker MN: Heinz Kohut's self-psychology: an overview. Am J Psychiatry 144:1–9, 1987

Beardslee WR: The role of self understanding in resilient individuals: the development of a perspective. Am J Orthopsychiatry 59:266–278, 1989

Benson H: The Relaxation Response. New York, William Morrow, 1975, pp 112–122

Berger B, Owen D: Anxiety reduction with swimming: relationship between exercise and state and trait anxiety. International Journal of Sport Psychology 18:286–302, 1987

Blair SN, Cole HW, Paffenbarger RS, et al: Physical fitness and all-cause mortality: a prospective study of healthy men and women. JAMA 262:2395–2401, 1989

Csikszentmihalyi M: Flow: The Psychology of Optimal Exercise. New York, Harper & Row, 1990

Donaldson BS: Strong Medicine. Garden City, NY, Doubleday, 1962

Druss RG, Silverman JA: The body image and perfectionism of ballerinas: comparison and contrast to anorexia nervosa. Gen Hosp Psychiatry 1:115–121, 1979

Dunbar C: The antihypertensive effects of exercise training. N Y State J Med 92:250–255, 1992

Emde R: Positive emotions for psychoanalytic theory: surprises from infancy research and new directions. J Am Psychoanal Assoc 39 (suppl):5–44, 1991

Freud S: The ego and the id (1923), in the Standard Edition of the Complete Psychological Works of Sigmund Freud, Vol 19. Translated and edited by Strachey J. London, Hogarth Press, 1962, pp 3–63

Glesser J, Mendelberg H: Exercise and sport in mental health: a review of the literature. Isr J Psychiatry Relat Sci 27:99–112, 1990

Greist JH, Eischens RR, Klein MH, et al: Antidepressant running. Psychiatric Annals 9:23–33, 1979

Holmes N, Cappo S: Prophylactic effect of aerobic fitness on cardiovascular arousal among individuals with a family history of hypertension. J Psychosom Res 31:601–605, 1987

Kobasa SC, Ouellette K, Puccetti MC: Personality and social resources in stress resistance. J Pers Soc Psychol 45:839–850, 1983

Krolner B, Taft B, Nielson SP: Physical exercise as a prophylaxis against involuntary bone loss: a controlled trial. Clin Sci 64:541–546, 1983

Lasch C: The Culture of Narcissism. New York, WW Norton, 1978

Lobstein D, Rasmussen C, Dunphy G, et al: Beta-endorphin and components of depression as powerful discriminators between joggers and sedentary middle-aged men. J Psychosom Res 33:291–305, 1989

Long B: Stress-management interventions: a 15-month follow-up of aerobic conditioning and stress modulation training. Cognitive Therapy Research 9:428–471, 1985

Long B, Haney C: Coping strategies for working women: aerobic exercise and relaxation instructions. Behav Ther 19:75–83, 1988

Morgan WP, Goldston SE: Summary, in Exercise and Mental Health. Edited by Morgan WP, Goldston SE. Washington, DC, Hemisphere, 1987, pp 3–7

O'Neill M: Unusual heart therapy wins coverage from large insurer. New York Times, July 28, 1993, p 1

Ornish D: Dean Ornish's Program for Reversing Heart Disease. New York, Random House, 1990, pp 323–349

Ossip-Klein DJ, Doyne EJ, Bowman ED, et al: Effects of running and weight lifting on self-concept in clinically depressed women. J Consult Clin Psychol 57:158–161, 1989

Paffenbarger RS, Wing AL, Hyde RT, et al: A natural history of athleticism and cardiovascular health. JAMA 252:491–495, 1984

Sacks MA: A psychoanalytic perspective on running, in Running as Therapy: An Integrated Approach. Edited by Sachs ML, Buffone G. Lincoln, University of Nebraska Press, 1984, pp 101–111

Sacks MA: Psychiatry and sport. Annals of Sports Medicine 5:47–52, 1990

Schwartz C: Exercise and anxiety disorders. Am J Psychiatry 146:1357–1358, 1989

Simons A, McGowan C, Epstein L, et al: Exercise as a treatment for depression: an update. Psychol Rev 5:553–568, 1985

Solomon E, Bumpers A: The running meditation response: an adjunct to psychotherapy. Am J Psychother 32:583–592, 1978

Taylor C, Houston-Miller N, Ahn D, et al: The effects of exercise training programs on psychosocial improvement in uncomplicated postmyocardial infarction patients. J Psychosom Res 30:581–587, 1986

Zinman B, Vranic M: Diabetes and exercise. Med Clin North Am 69:145–157, 1985

Index